How to Develop Your Career in Dentistry

How to Develop Your Career in Dentistry

Janine Brooks MBE, DMed Eth, MSc, FFGDPUK, MCDH, DDPHRCS, FAcadMed, BDS

Dentalia Coaching & Training Consultancy

WILEY Blackwell

This edition first published 2015 © 2015 by John Wiley & Sons Ltd.

Registered office: John Wiley & Sons, Ltd, The Atrium, Southern Gate, Chichester, West Sussex, PO19 8SQ, UK

Editorial offices: 9600 Garsington Road, Oxford, OX4 2DQ, UK
  The Atrium, Southern Gate, Chichester, West Sussex, PO19 8SQ, UK
  1606 Golden Aspen Drive, Suites 103 and 104, Ames, Iowa 50010, USA

For details of our global editorial offices, for customer services and for information about how to apply for permission to reuse the copyright material in this book please see our website at www.wiley.com/wiley-blackwell

The right of the author to be identified as the author of this work has been asserted in accordance with the UK Copyright, Designs and Patents Act 1988.

Library of Congress Cataloging-in-Publication Data

Brooks, Janine, author.
  How to develop your career in dentistry / Janine Brooks.
    p. ; cm.
  Includes bibliographical references and index.
  ISBN 978-1-118-91381-9 (pbk.)
  I. Title.
  [DNLM: 1. Dentistry–Great Britain. 2. Vocational Guidance–Great Britain. WU 21]
  RK60
  617.6′0232–dc23

                                                         2015015317

A catalogue record for this book is available from the British Library.

Wiley also publishes its books in a variety of electronic formats. Some content that appears in print may not be available in electronic books.

Set in 9.5/12 pt MinionPro by SPi Global, Chennai, India
Printed and bound in Malaysia by Vivar Printing Sdn Bhd

1   2015

Contents

Chapter 3   Dental opportunities, 57

Chapter 4   Coaching and mentoring, 99

Chapter 5   Case studies of dental professionals, 118

Chapter 6   Networking and networks, 150

Foreword

As someone who many might say reached the top of a dental career pathway, I think it is really interesting to look back and analyse what the principle drivers were in that career.

Developing a successful career involves a range of skills and an ability to be analytical in assessing the needs of the population, ignoring high-profile commercial pressures and learning where to get objective and constructive advice and criticism.

I think it is fundamental to understand that change is a constant and not to see change as a challenge but as an opportunity. An unreasonable commitment to the status quo is unlikely to lead to a successful career.

The significance of change and the need to treat it as an opportunity is true whether we are talking about a purely clinical career, be that in specialties or in general practice (and I think that differentiation will blur more and more in the coming years), the development of services or the area of public health.

The oral health of the nation has improved dramatically during my career, as have patient expectations and clinical techniques.

Ultimately, to feel fulfilled during your career you need to feel you have played your part in improving services to patients and have used your skills to the full.

A quality service, on both macro and micro scales, is one which is safe, clinically effective and makes the patient feel they have been treated with respect.

Key to the delivery of this aim is the development of high-quality clinical and professional leadership, and using your clinical skills and knowledge to improve services and outcomes for patients is one of the most rewarding things you can do. I would urge readers to take note of the advice in this book, which is written by someone who has a good knowledge of education and leadership.

Barry Cockcroft CBE
Chief Dental Officer for England
2006–2015

Acknowledgements

I have been incredibly fortunate to have received contributions from a number of talented dental professionals, who between them demonstrate a huge range of the roles and responsibilities available to us in dentistry. They have generously written their career stories and shared their CVs with me and allowed me to pester them frequently for information. I am very grateful to them all, and I believe their words make careers in dentistry more accessible. As role models, they are second to none.

List of contributors

Jackie Arnold
Geraldine Birks
Malcolm Brady
Steve Boyle
Steve Brookes
Helen Caton-Hughes (for permission to use the 'Forton Transformational Coaching 4-Quadrant Diagram')
Bal Chana
Manish Chitnis
Janet Clarke MBE
Jane Dalgarno
Jane Davies-Slowik
Ken Eaton
Sara Holmes MBE
Ros Keaton
Estelle Los
Grainee Lynn (for checking accuracy)
Shazad Malik
Penny McWilliams
Margaret Nash
Sophie Noske

Reena Patel
Claudia Peace
Nichola Peasnell
Keith Percival
Heather Pope
Derek Richards
Ian Taylor
David Thomas (for checking accuracy)
Peter Thornley
Deborah White
Emma Worrell

I am also extremely grateful to a non-dental professional who has also contributed so generously of his time: John Brooks, my husband. He has tirelessly proof read the manuscript and offered a much needed sense check, allowing me to see the wood for the trees.

Chapter 1 **Introduction**

```
                                    Y
T  O              N                 O
E        D        U        D        U
C  A  R  E  E  R  S        E  X  P  E  R  T
H        N        S        V
N        T        E        D  E  N  T  I  S  T
I        I  N              L
C        S                 O
I        T     H  E  R  A  P  I  S  T
A        R
N        H  Y  G  I  E  N  I  S  T
                                 H  O  W
```

> **Top Tip:** *Don't be afraid to tack – take the nonlinear path*
>
> Janine Brooks

Welcome to my book on *How to Develop your Career in Dentistry*. I hope you find it interesting and useful. I hope it makes you think about your career and encourages you to dip your toes into an exciting world of diversity and opportunity.

The approach I want to take is that our careers can be multistranded: I'm calling that having a 'portfolio career'. In addition, I want to get you to think about the context in which we provide dentistry, our Society. Chapter 2 covers changes happening within society that will impact on dental professionals and the career choices they make. These include changes to retirement and pensions, as well as demographic changes, particularly in health and longevity, both of our patients and of us dental professionals. Chapter 3 discusses dental opportunities; here I will be giving you a taster of the many roles and responsibilities that dental professionals take on. Chapter 4 is about mentoring and coaching, both of which I feel are essential support for dental professionals seeking development and career enhancement. Chapter 5 I have dedicated to case studies. I have been fortunate in

---

How to Develop Your Career in Dentistry, First Edition. Janine Brooks.
© 2015 John Wiley & Sons, Ltd. Published 2015 by John Wiley & Sons, Ltd.

persuading a number of dental professionals to share their career stories with me and to allow me to include them in this book. I feel this is the heart of the book, as it showcases the breadth and depth of dental professionals' talents. Chapter 6 covers networking and networks: again, in my opinion, essential to a successful career. Finally, Chapter 7 discusses training and the qualifications you may want to think about when enriching your career and expanding what you do. Throughout the book, I have sprinkled Top Tips – both my own and those of other professionals. Feel free to give them a go. They may not all work for you, but some will. I have also sprinkled Career Highlights from a number of contributors throughout the chapters. To me, they demonstrate that dentistry is very rewarding and that, even if we struggle and find the demands of others a challenge, there is plenty of light and plenty of rewards to keep us going.

> *The self is not something ready made, but something in continuous formation, through choice of action.*

> Dewey (1916)

I really like this quote from Dewey. When he wrote it, he was thinking about reflection, but I feel it is very relevant to making choices and building a career. Opportunities may arise unexpectedly and unplanned, and often from the strangest direction, but it is our choice what action we take – no one else's. Take control, be the architect of your career. This may mean taking a few 'risks', maybe doing something for free. Make it part of your plan to be more opportunistic. If you learn to translate what you see, hear and do into your career, you might be surprised by the shape it takes on.

Career Highlight: *Voluntary work abroad*

Reena Patel

Another important aspect of the Dewey quote for me is the word 'continuous'. Our careers should be continuous, growing, expanding, evolving, not static or stale. In dentistry, we are fortunate in being part of a profession that has a rich diversity of jobs and roles. I'm not saying it's easy, I'm not saying there won't be strong competition for some of the jobs you want, but you worked hard to enter the profession – that you need to work hard to build your career should not be a surprise.

Our career takes up a large proportion of our middle life – that's the life between leaving school (largely childhood) and retiring (largely older age). It obviously varies from person to person, but as a very rough estimate you will spend a minimum of 2775 full days (24 hours of each day – no sleeping) or 66 600 hours working. That will hold if the following are true:

- You leave school at 18 years.
- You spend 5 years training in your primary qualification.
- You retire at 60 years of age.
- You work 5 days a week, and take no time off for your family.
- You take 6 weeks' annual leave each year.
- You are sick for 5 days each year.

As you can see, this is a very rough estimate, based on variables that have considerable range. If you start work earlier, have less training time, retire earlier or later, work part time or take time off to raise your family, have less annual leave and are particularly healthy then you will spend even longer in your career. It's very likely most people reading this book will not retire at 60 years of age.

The real point I'm making here is that you will spend a considerable amount of your life working in your career. I guess that doesn't come as a surprise. What might, though, is exactly how much time it is. Until you really think about it, you probably just consider it 'a lot'. So, if you are going to spend 'a lot' of your life tending to your career then the least you can do for yourself is make choices that you will enjoy and find fulfilling and satisfying. The good news is that the profession of dentistry can offer exactly that, plus a good remuneration – maybe not the best, but good nonetheless. Of course, you may be looking for a career where you do very little, make loads of money and have lots of spare time. If you are, then stop reading this book immediately: dentistry is not for you. Look for something else. Please don't ask my advice on what that something else might be: I hate being bored.

> **Career Highlight:** *The launch of the* Evidence-Based Dentistry *journal*
> Derek Richards

Just before I get into the meat of careers in dentistry and developing your dental career, I want to take a few words to consider where dentistry has come from and our origins as dental professionals. Don't worry, this is not an essay on history, just some interesting context. I think it can be useful to look back and consider where dentistry and dental professionals have come from before we look forward to the careers of the future. Dentistry has a very long history: the practice of dentistry much more so than the professions. All aspects are fascinating and serve to underline what is an amazing career for those who choose it.

There are a number of books and authors in this field far better equipped than I to paint and illustrate this history. In particular, I would direct you to the excellent articles and publications of Professor Stanley Gelbier, a tireless and exceptionally knowledgeable dental historian. I wish to use our history to put our careers in dentistry into context, so I will only whet your appetite, and signpost your way should you wish to delve more deeply.

A good place to begin would be to define dentistry. Some early cultures mutilated their teeth: whether as decoration or to denote religious status or perhaps to intimidate others is uncertain. Whatever the true purpose, someone will have worked on these teeth: Is that dentistry? We know the Egyptians practised dentistry: the Ptolemic temple at Kom Ombo (north of Aswan), the temple of Sobek and Horus, has a huge wall with wonderful carvings depicting surgical instruments, including forceps (Figure 1.1).

In the British Isles, those who would eventually become the dentists we know today were once part of the Guild of Barber-Surgeons, created in 1540. Most of those who engaged in 'dentistry' in the 16th century identified themselves with the barber surgeons rather than the physicians; that is why dentists in the UK have historically referred to themselves as 'Mister' or 'Miss' rather than as 'Doctor'. Dentistry did not generally take the same path outside of Britain. The Guild broke apart in 1745, when the Surgeons'

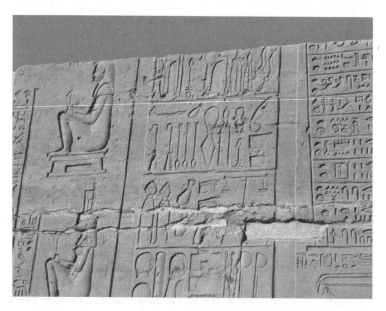

Figure 1.1 Kom Ombo wall, north of Aswan, showing 2000-year-old surgical instruments. Taken by the author in February 2012.

Company was formed; that company later dissolved in 1796 and then reformed as the Royal College of Surgeons of England in 1800. The barbers, dentists and 'operators for the teeth' took a different path, although a few barbers and tooth-drawers went with the Royal College. Eventually, the term 'dentist' became the accepted and acceptable term by which to encompass all these previous descriptors.

Moving through the years, we come to the Dentist Act of 1878 and the first UK dental register of 1879. Dentists had previously been included in the medical register: the edition of 1783 included 18 (Bishop, 2014). In 1921, there was another Dentist Act. The Dental Board (UK) of the General Medical Council was established and its first Chairman, Sir Francis Dyke Acland, was appointed by the Privy Council. When the Board was established, there were 5831 names on the register. The first regulation of dentists was by the medical profession. This continued until 1956, when the General Dental Council (GDC) was established as a standalone regulator. The 70th and final session of the Dental Board was held on 9 May 1956 and the first meeting of the GDC took place later in the same year, both under the chairmanship of Sir Wilfred Fish. At that time, in 1956, there were 15 895 names on the dental register, all dentists, and the dental schools had an entry of 650 students each year. I am indebted to a little book I found on a visit to the bookshops of Hay-on-Wye for this fascinating insight into the history of the profession in the United Kingdom (Dental Board of the UK (1957)).

> **Career Highlight:** *Undertaking and completing a PhD*
>
> Debbie White

In 1858, the Dental Hospital of London opened as the first clinical training school for dentists in the United Kingdom. Dental Schools began to open soon afterwards. Previously, dentists were trained as apprentices by more experienced dentists. In 1860, the first licences of dental surgery were awarded by the Royal College of Surgeons of England. The first dental degree was awarded by the University of Birmingham in 1901. Non-dentist dental professionals, with the exception of dental technicians, joined the ranks of the dental team a little later.

Dental therapists made an appearance in 1917 as 'dental dressers' in some English counties. This is probably earlier than you might think. Their role was based on that of American hygienists, although British dressers could also fill teeth that had no pulpal involvement and extract deciduous teeth. They were the early dental therapists. In 1960, New Cross Hospital began training dental auxiliaries (British Association of Dental Therapists).

The British Dental Nurses and Assistants Society was established in 1940 by Madeleine Winter, a dental nurse, and her dentist, Mr P. Grundy. They worked in Leyland, Lancashire. However, formal training for dental nurses did not begin until the 1930s. This organisation has become the British Association of Dental Nurses (BADN).

Dental hygienists emerged in 1943 when the Women's Auxiliary Air Force began to offer training. The first British dental hygienists qualified in 1944.

The history of dental technology and dental technicians is founded in antiquity. Dental appliances belonging to the Etruscans (in Italy) have been found from the middle of the 7th century BC (Becker, 1999). In 1728, one 'Gamaliel Voice' of Whalebone Court, Lothby was selling dentures by mail order in England (Royal College of Dental Surgeons of Ontario, 1889). Today, dental technology has a number of branches:

- prosthodontic technicians;
- conservation technicians;
- orthodontic technicians; and
- maxillofacial technicians (sometimes also known as maxillofacial prosthetists).

Our newest professional groups are orthodontic therapists and clinical dental technicians. Registration with the GDC for both groups became open from 1999. The first training course for orthodontic therapists started in Leeds in July 2007. The British Orthodontic Society (2011) has published a fascinating history of the events leading up to the establishment of orthodontic therapists in the United Kingdom, beginning in October 1967.

For clinical dental technicians, the story is an interesting evolution from the term 'denturist'. Laws allowing the supply of dentures to the public without the intervention of a dentist have been passed in 11 countries across the globe, including the United Kingdom in 2007. Clinical dental technicians have now joined the family of dental registrants (International Federation of Denturists, 2013).

> **Top Tip:** *Never give up – you will make it to the top*
>
> Shazad Malik

The National Health Service

Whether you decide to work directly within the National Health Service (NHS) or not, it will have an impact on your career. Since its creation on 5 July 1948, the NHS has become an essential ingredient of the culture of the United Kingdom. As Figure 1.2 demonstrates, the NHS is one of those aspects of Britishness of which people are most proud.

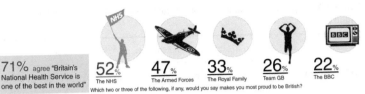

71% agree "Britain's National Health Service is one of the best in the world"

52% The NHS

47% The Armed Forces

33% The Royal Family

26% Team GB

22% The BBC

Which two or three of the following, if any, would you say makes you most proud to be British?

Figure 1.2 Sources of British pride. Source: Ipsos MORI 2013. Making sense of society, NHS at 65. https://www.ipsos-mori.com/newsevents/blogs/makingsenseofsociety/1553/Maintaining-pride-in-the-NHS-The-challenge-for-the-new-NHS-Chief-Exec.aspx#gallery[m]/0/ (last accessed 18 March 2015).

The founding principle of medical, dental, optical and pharmaceutical care free at the point of access was broken within a few short years of the birth of the NHS, largely by the public need for dentures and spectacles. On 1 June 1952, a flat rate of £1 for ordinary dental care was introduced and charges were made for dentures (House of Commons Health Committee, 2006). Then, as now, there were insufficient resources to meet the health needs of the population. That aside, the majority of dental professionals work in the NHS at some point in their career, and even those who are wholly private will be impacted by NHS principles of governance. The numerous reorganisations of the NHS have shaped the careers of everyone working in or alongside it for over 30 years, and it is likely that they will continue to do so for the next 30 years or more.

Today, every English dental professional will have cause to come into contact with the following four organisations to a greater or lesser extent: NHS England, Public Health England, the Care Quality Commission (CQC) (responsible for the quality of dental practices) and Monitor (responsible for overall market regulation). Between them, these organisations are responsible for the health of the English community, through direct provision and governance. Table 1.1 lists the equivalent organisations for Wales, Scotland and Northern Ireland.

Top Tip: Be flexible

Debbie White

Career Highlight: Receiving, when I was leaving Worcestershire, very many cards, letters and e-mails from colleagues, staff, patients and carers thanking me for what I had done. A highly affirming experience

Ros Keeton

Table 1.1 Organisations that impact on dental professions in the United Kingdom, by country

England	Northern Ireland	Scotland	Wales
NHS England	Health & Social Care Board Dept. of Health, Social Services & Public Safety Business Services Organisation	NHS Scotland	Local Health Boards as part of NHS Wales
Public Health England	Public Health Agency	NHS National Service, Scotland	Public Health Wales
Care Quality Commission	Regulation and Quality Improvement Authority (private dentists)	Healthcare Improvement Scotland	Healthcare Inspectorate Wales
Monitor			

Career

So, having set a little of the scene in which our profession has been founded and in which it operates today, I want to begin to turn to the meat of the book: developing your career in dentistry. What is a career? The word has a Latin origin: it means, 'to go around the ancient Roman racetrack at top speed in a precipitous headlong rush'. Somehow I don't find that particularly helpful for the modern day, although it may be for some people that their career does seem akin to a precipitous headlong rush. Other definitions are available.

The Oxford English Reference Dictionary (Oxford University Press, 1996) describes 'career' as 'One's advancement through life, especially in a profession'. In this definition, 'career' is understood to relate to a range of aspects of an individual's life, learning and work. 'Career' is also frequently understood to relate to the working aspects of an individual's life, as in 'career woman', for example.

Another way in which the term 'career' is used is to 'describe an occupation or a profession that usually involves special training or formal education, and is considered to be a person's lifework' (Oxford University Press, 1996). In this case a 'career' is seen as a sequence of related jobs usually pursued within a single industry or sector; for example, 'a career in law' or 'a career in the building trade', or, in our case, 'a career in dentistry'.

The second definition seems to fit with a dental career. Interestingly, it refers to a sequence of related jobs rather than to one specific job for the lifetime of the career. This seems to represent a linear progression. However, I do like the idea of a career being about progress through life and relating to a range of aspects of life. For me, that seems to fit nicely with a portfolio: a more diverse way of looking at our work. It also fits with sometimes stepping outside a specific industry, so dental professionals stepping out of dentistry or indeed stepping out of the health sector would be accommodated in this definition.

> **Top Tip:** *Make yourself visible – speak up*
>
> Reena Patel

In this book, I intend to consider what a career in dentistry might mean in the widest and deepest possible way. I will cover the more well known aspects of clinical dentistry in general practice, salaried services and secondary care, as well as the less well known roles dental professional undertake. These will include both clinical and nonclinical work. I also intend to be inclusive of all dental registrants, and not just dentists. This book will be of interest and, I hope, use to all those registered with the GDC, those who are training to become a dental professional and maybe even those who are still to make up their mind about whether dentistry is the profession for them. Finally, overseas dental professionals might find the information helpful if they are thinking about working in the United Kingdom.

If we define a career as an occupation or profession with a sequence of related jobs, usually pursued within a single industry or sector, we can think of dentistry as the profession and health services as the sector. That can be interesting when we are thinking about developing our career over a lifetime of work. Figure 1.3 illustrates movement between occupations and sectors. It would work equally well should we want to step out of dentistry into a completely new occupation. An example might be dental professionals who have become trust chief executives or who have moved into law. As with most models, it can be adapted to help you think about your specific environment and your specific choices.

> **Top Tip:** *You've one life, so enjoy every day*
>
> Emma Worrell

It seems that people in work today are more likely to experience a number of career changes during their lives than we once were. That might be complete retraining (e.g. a dental professional retraining to become a lawyer) or a change of direction within dentistry (e.g. becoming a tutor). The actual

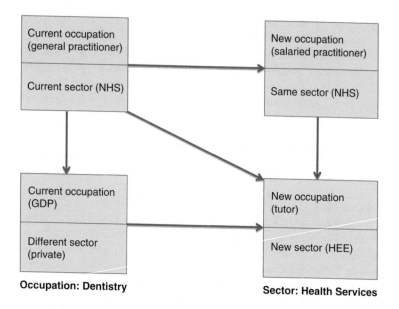

Figure 1.3 Model illustrating moving between sectors and occupations.

number of career changes an individual will make can vary: it might be three, it might be six or even more. On the whole, Baby Boomers are happiest with stability, while members of Generation Y are more likely to be job jumpers. Whatever the number, what is more relevant is the concept of job jumping. I suspect, as people start to work longer before retirement, we are likely to see more career changes in the future. Let me clarify what I mean by 'career changes': I mean broadening what you do, so taking on more part-time responsibilities could be just as much a career change as taking on a completely new job. If you think of dentistry as a pie, and general practice as apple pie, then why have apple pie for the whole of your life? Why not have some plum pie or rhubarb pie or beef and ale pie? Why not enliven your career with lots of different flavours? We don't eat exactly the same food for our whole life, so why would we keep exactly the same job?

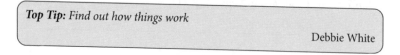

Top Tip: Find out how things work

Debbie White

Mark Savickas (Savickas *et al.*, 2009) talks of 'life trajectories'. He suggests that people actively design and build their lives progressively, including their working careers. This makes perfect sense to me: people should use their skills and experience to take the next step in their career. This could include practical skills and experience, as well as learnt or taught skills. A mixing of experience with new knowledge. I think that's what experienced dental professionals do as they build a portfolio career. Sometimes you might acquire a new skill or knowledge that doesn't seem to be immediately useful in your life trajectory. You might be surprised to find that as you move a little further into the matrix of your career that that skill is just what you need to take on something you really want to do. I found this to be true when I took on being Data Protection Manager for my Trust, then local Caldicott Guardian, and later found it prepared me for becoming the NHS Information Authority Caldicott Guardian. That was my first national job and it prepared me for other national jobs and taking my career into unexpected but exciting waters. When it comes to acquiring experience and skills, most can be recycled and not much is wasted if you are prepared to be creative and imaginative, or maybe just to take a few calculated risks.

Savickas teamed up with Donald and Charles Super (Super *et al.*, 1996) to introduce his approach of *life span, life space* to career choice and development. Savickas, Super and Super suggest that:

> *The new job market in our unsettled economy calls for viewing career not as a lifetime commitment to one employer but as selling services and skills to a series of employers who need projects completed. In negotiating each new project, the prospective employee usually concentrates on salary yet also seeks to make the work meaningful, control the work environment, balance work-family responsibilities, and train for the next job.*

This underpins a portfolio career that includes a number of employers or projects. It also introduces a variety of factors that influence which new roles or projects we might take on. Money is a factor, but only one of a number. In developing your portfolio, it may be that for you the more important factor is making work more meaningful or acquiring skills for the next job. Savickas, Super and Super also write about a career as being cyclical, with five stages: growth, exploration, establishment, maintenance and disengagement. Interestingly, they write about mini-cycles, in which we go through the same stages several times within our complete career. This fits with a career as a series of projects. I rather like the way this model can be applied to the careers available to dental professionals. We go through the five stages over our career lifetime in dentistry as we train (growth), try out a few jobs in our first few years (exploration), consolidate our skills and experience (establishment), keep ourselves up to date and on an even keel (maintenance) and finally phase out of working (disengagement). You can

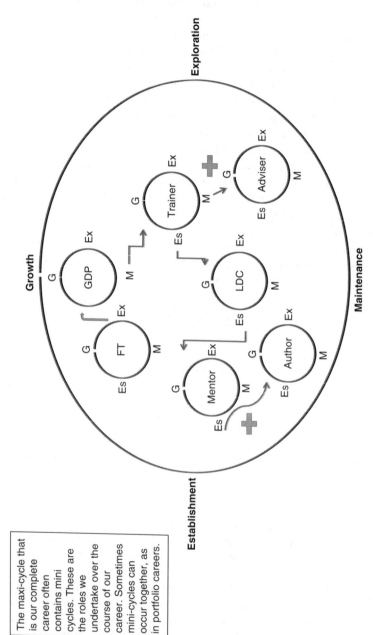

The maxi-cycle that is our complete career often contains mini cycles. These are the roles we undertake over the course of our career. Sometimes mini-cycles can occur together, as in portfolio careers.

Figure 1.4 Career cycles (adapted from Super et al., 1996).

also see how this applies to mini-cycles for specific jobs or responsibilities: one person working through several mini-cycles while the maxi-cycle of their working life continues. A model of wheels/circles within wheels/circles is revealed. Applying that model to a portfolio career works well. I have included my own adaptation of the model and put in dental examples so you can see how it works for a portfolio career.

> **Top Tip:** *Read about people whose achievements inspire you – they've over-come far greater hurdles than you*
>
> Reena Patel

Portfolio career

What do I mean by 'portfolio'? It has many meanings, which is quite appropriate, really. It can be a collection of assets – buildings, stocks and shares, cash – but that's not what I mean. It can be a collection of electronic documents – that's also not what I mean. It can be an organised collection of education, skills or experiences – still, not really what I mean. What I mean is something that has a number of strands or threads; something multistranded, if you will. What about a portfolio career? That would be a career that has many strands, threads or aspects. That means there is no such thing as one portfolio career. It's not something you can apply for: you won't see a job advertisement for a portfolio career. Portfolio careers are unique, special, yours. You create your portfolio, a personalised career. Brilliant: you can build in all the things you enjoy doing, all the things you are good at – how great is that? I see a variety of portfolios, ranging from more than one job in the same sector, perhaps more than one general practice position, to a career package that extends to several jobs across a number of sectors of dentistry, health care and beyond. There is no one portfolio career: there are as many as the people who have them – thousands, probably millions. My feeling is that while different jobs in the same sector hit the spot for increased interest, for maximum diversity, sector mixing or blending makes for a true portfolio. A good portfolio *is* the career. It's not trying out things while you wait for the big opportunity; it *is* the big opportunity.

Before this term was used widely, I considered myself to be a 'ticket collector'. By that I mean I actively sought out new responsibilities and new jobs, so when I was offered the chance to manage a cottage hospital or other professional group, or to project manage a merger or the Year 2000 project, or to be data protection manager or Caldicott Guardian, I said yes. You might think, 'Bully for you, I'm a dentist, I treat patients, you can leave that other stuff, thank you'. My point is there isn't anything I have done that didn't give me new skills, didn't help me be a better dentist and didn't help me stay fresh and enthusiastic about my career. I benefitted, my patients benefitted and those around me benefitted. A win, win, win situation.

> **Top Tip:** *Always follow your dreams*
>
> Sophie Noske

Of course, as with anything, there are advantages and disadvantages, good things and not so good things. On the positive side:
- There are so many interesting 'small' things you can do.
- You can take on new things.
- You choose what you do.
- Your time is your own to organise – if you want mornings free, take them.
- You take full responsibility for what you do (nothing new there for dental professionals).
- It's hard work – don't you just love hard work (when it's for you)?
- You are not reliant on a single income stream.
- There is always something new.

On the slightly less great side:
- It's hard work – not a walk in the park.
- You take full responsibility for what you do – no one else to blame – no buck passing.
- There will be fluctuations in income stream.
- There is a lack of stability.
- You need to be a good organiser (that might be a positive thing as well).

I think you can see that some things can be viewed as positive and negative at the same time: it depends on how you see them. I love working hard and taking responsibility. Don't think about a portfolio career if you're basically a lazy person who likes things given to you on a plate. Actually, I can't really see you in dentistry if you're that type of person.

Most people will begin their portfolio from a base: one regular income stream, maybe one that takes up 2–3 days a week. You can then begin to build and add new streams.

I think of a portfolio as a portfolio life rather than just a career: mixing it all up, blending and creating your life as you go – why not, why be constrained by boundaries? The important thing about a portfolio life is that it's right for you.

> **Career Highlight:** *Being made a professor*
>
> Debbie White

Working paradigms

Paradigms denote or describe patterns of what is accepted. Working paradigms are typical examples, so if we think of the paradigm of career patterns then we can think of the old and then the new patterns for careers. In Table 1.2, I list some aspects of the old and the new working paradigms. The changes can be thought of as representing a paradigm shift in our thinking about the components of an accepted career.

The old patterns saw a career as a single pathway; for example, the general practitioner who remained a general practitioner, often in the same practice, for the whole of his or her working life: a full-time clinician providing a service for their group of patients. Eventually, at 60 or 65 years of age, they would retire and move from full-time worker to full-time nonworker. This was seen as steady, the norm for the majority. Sometimes, they might have moved to a different practice, but the pattern was one of little change. The new pattern of working is quite different: the new practitioner moves both geographically and between aspects of dentistry. Those who remain within one sector often take on other responsibilities, usually while retaining a clinical commitment, which might reduce over the years to make room for other roles and responsibilities. Their career tacks around, sometimes with a move upwards, sometimes with a move sideways and sometimes with a move a few steps back. The ladder has been replaced by the climbing frame (Figures 1.5 and 1.6). These practitioners manage their careers and, rather than wait for organisations to offer opportunities, they make their own opportunities. The shift from the old patterns to the new has been taking place for some years now, as more and more people find the new ways of working more rewarding and are prepared to take risks with their career choices.

> **Top Tip:** *Everything is achievable, never give up*
>
> Bal Chana

Table 1.2 Moving from old paradigms to new ways of working

Paradigm shift $\longrightarrow$	
Old	New
Stable, little change	Constant, rapid change
Little movement between jobs	More movement
Straight-line progression	Matrix, climbing frame
Organisation looks after you	You manage your career
Stress	Stress
Single role/job	Multiple roles/jobs
Retirement	Phased

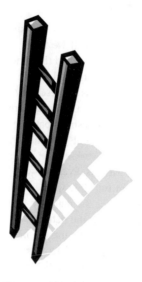

Figure 1.5 Out with the old …

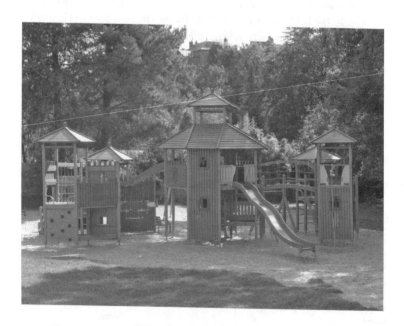

Figure 1.6 … In with the new.

Some people talk about a good career as one in which they can climb up, one job at a time, until they rise to the top, the pinnacle of success. As they climb, the jobs get fewer and fewer, until they have achieved the single top job. Some career pathways still look like that: we still talk about the 'career ladder'. In essence, the old career pattern was that you stayed with a single job all your working life and you progressed until you had reached the top: usually a position of seniority from which you would retire to a full-time life at home; a one-way street.

The new career pattern is one of change, changing jobs, changing sectors, moving around, maybe with some time overseas. You gain more experience and skills, taking on different roles, perhaps several part-time, some voluntary, and you manage your life to include home and work in a balance that works for you and your family. Retirement is rarely full-time but becomes a phased blurring, with perhaps more time working from home and a slow transition from more to less work.

Those dental professionals who register with the GDC in 2015 can probably expect to work until 2060 – a career of 45 years – with formal retirement at a minimum of 68 years and maybe even later than that. That's a very long time to remain on a single pathway. Those dental professionals currently working can look forward to increasing changes: some exciting, some scary and most in between. The predictions I introduce in this book, particularly in relation to the age and health of the population, will take account of the next 40–45 years.

It's my experience that dentistry is a diverse and fascinating career, and I'm writing this book to share the opportunities available for all dental professionals. It's my hope that the information you find here will give you inspiration to broaden your career and help you find out more about those aspects of dentistry you may know little about. When I began training at Birmingham Dental School I had already had a career in Medical Laboratory Technology. I left school at 16 and became a trainee laboratory technician at Aston University. Later, I moved to work in Haematology and Cytogenetics at East Birmingham Hospital (now Heartlands Hospital). By the time I entered dental school, I was a mature student, albeit only 24 years old. I had also been married. In those days, Birmingham was keen to admit a few students each year with 'nontraditional' entry requirements. Perhaps I have always been attracted to being 'nontraditional'. I find life far too interesting to get locked on to a single path stretching endlessly ahead. I developed a portfolio career way before I knew this was what I was doing. I knew I enjoyed variety and found juggling a number of jobs/roles energising. During my career in dentistry I have found I'm not alone in enjoying diversity: many colleagues combine a large number of aspects of dentistry within their career. Several of those inspiring dental professionals have generously shared their curriculum vitaes and career histories with me so that I can share them with you. This book both looks broadly and dives deeply. It looks at individuals who have achieved the portfolio and enjoy a variety of roles within their working week, month and year. But it also dives deep into specific career opportunities to tell you more about the realities of each part of dentistry. Colleagues from all aspects of dentistry have shared what they do, what they like best and what they like least.

> **Top Tip:** *There is almost always more than one solution to a problem*
>
> Derek Richards

Planning your career

You made it: you've qualified as a dental professional. So, that's it, right? Wrong. Dentistry is not one career, it's a multitude of careers. You don't know what you don't know, so how can you find out what's available? How can you decide what's for you, what you might enjoy and be good at? I'm hopeful that this book will answer some of those questions, and signpost and open doors so that you can find out the rest.

One thing you do need is to understand yourself and what excites you, what you feel passionate about, what makes you get up in the morning. Those are the things that push you and motivate you. You could think of those 'push' factors as being made up of:

- home/family (H);
- yourself (Y); and
- work (W).

You can construct a visual image of these important motivators using a simple pie chart (Figure 1.7). You might want to think about the size of each of the portions and whether one is larger or smaller than the others. I would not

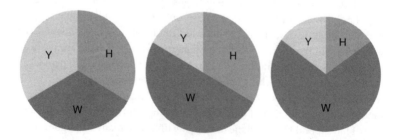

Figure 1.7 Push factors.

presume to suggest aiming for one particular pie chart over the others, only that you think about how your own life is divided and which is the right balance for you. It doesn't matter if it's not the same as everyone else's, just that it suits you.

> **Top Tip:** *Be interested in people*
>
> Debbie White

Somewhere along the line of development we discover what we really are, and then we make our real decision, for which we are responsible. Make that decision primarily for yourself because you can never really live anyone else's life

Eleanor Roosevelt

In 1994, Brousseau and Driver developed a career concept model in which they suggested different types of careers and how people described their ideal careers (Figure 1.8). The Linear career travels in one direction, generally upwards, taking on more responsibility and authority as it goes until it reaches the top. Of course, it can also represent those who remain in the same job in the same grade for their whole working life – in which case, the line is a horizontal one. The Expert chooses their career field and sticks with it. Typically, health professionals take this career route. The person is the career: you are a dentist, or a dental technician, or a dental nurse, rather than

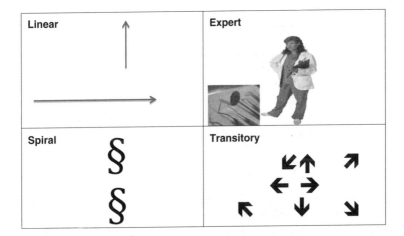

Figure 1.8 Career types and ideal careers (Brousseau and Driver, 1994).

working in dentistry. The Spiral route this is less traditional than the Linear or Expert. The person with a Spiral career enjoys major changes, perhaps moving from one field to another. This is my career pattern, although I was not aware of it for some time. Looking back, it seems so obvious. Finally, there is the Transitory career, which is the least traditional of the four. There is a considerable amount of change, in both jobs and career fields. The direction can be up, down, sideways or diagonal. It can appear quite chaotic. I have a sneaking suspicion there is an element of the Transitory in my career as well. Of course, our careers can be mixtures – we don't have to rigidly stick to one pattern.

> **Top Tip:** *Do not be afraid to try different things*
>
> Derek Richards

Careers in the future are more likely to take a Spiral or a Transitory route, even for the Expert professional. Each of the shapes of career described offers different rewards. For example, the model suggests that Linear careers are most strongly linked to power and achievement. Experts have a strong competence motive, with a high need for security and stability. Spiral careers offer personal growth and creativity, with highly individualistic career paths. Transitory careers involve lots of change, so they appeal to people who are motivated by novelty and value independence and immediate results.

> **Top Tip:** *Take opportunities (always)*
>
> Janine Brooks

You may want to give this model some thought if you feel you and your career are rather mismatched. The good news is that dentistry can offer career paths that take all these shapes, you just need to know which is most suited to you. Your career may begin as one type (e.g. Expert) and then become another (e.g. Spiral and then Linear for a while). Some aspects of your career may take the characteristics of one type and some aspects another.

Being a dental professional

Dentistry is not a particularly large profession. In December 2013, there were a total of just over 105 000 practitioners registered with the GDC across all seven registrant groups. Non-dentist registrants have been placed together as dental care professionals (DCPs) in Tables 1.3–1.5.

Table 1.3 Number of dentist GDC registrants (31.12.13)

Registration type	Count
Dental care professional	63 040
Dentist	40 424
Temporary registrant dentist	1671
Total	**105 135**

Source: General Dental Council.

Table 1.4 Number of DCP GDC registrants (31.12.13)

DCP type	Count
Clinical dental technician	234
Dental hygienist	6333
Dental nurse	50 651
Dental technician	6320
Dental therapist	2230
Orthodontic therapist	323
Total	**66 091**

Source: General Dental Council.

Table 1.5 Number of general dental practices (2013)

Country	Number of general dental practices
England	10 130
Scotland	1091
Northern Ireland	396
Wales	503
Total	**12 120**

Source: Care Quality Commission (2013).

Interestingly, there is a different total number of DCPs in the registrant type to the breakdown of DCPs. This may be due to double counting, as some DCPs will be registered under more than one professional category.

In England and Wales, practices are tendered for, so the ability to set up a new NHS practice is constrained. In Scotland and Northern Ireland, dentists retain the ability to establish new practices, and the number of practices has risen each year.

Top Tip: *Think about how you act, speak and look*

Reena Patel

Table 1.6 Relative numbers of dentists per English practice

Number of dentists	Proportion of practices (% of total)
1	19
2	17
3	15
4	12
5	10
6+	26

Source: Care Quality Commission (2013).

Almost one in five practices in England has only one dental practitioner (Table 1.6). Just over a quarter have a minimum of six dentists. Most dentists in 2013 worked in an environment with two to five dental colleagues. Unfortunately, working numbers of other dental professionals per practice are not available.

> **Top Tip:** *Have a good work ethic*
>
> Debbie White

Numbers in Wales and Northern Ireland are small, so the results should be treated with caution. However, Table 1.7 clearly shows the prevalence of

Table 1.7 General dental practices (BDA members 2013)

Practice type	UK	England	Wales	Northern Ireland	Scotland
Limited company	22.2	21.15	35.7%	20.0%	23.3%
Limited liability partnership	1.6	1.7%	0.0%	4.0%	1.4%
Partnership agreement	18.0	16.9%	19.0%	24.0%	23.3%
Sole trader with associates	32.2	31.6%	23.8%	40.0%	38.4%
Sole trader without associates	12.4	13.8%	11.9%	4.0%	5.5%
Expense sharing agreement	11.1	12.3%	7.1%	0.0%	8.2%
Other	2.5	2.6%	2.4%	8.0%	0.0%
Total percentage	**100%**	**100%**	**100%**	**100%**	**100%**
Total number	**684**	**544**	**42**	**25**	**73**

Source: BDA, Dental Business Trends, 2013.

dental companies. Nearly a quarter of associates work for a dental company. This may not be one of the large chains, but their importance in the dental arena is growing.

Corporate bodies tend to be more prevalent in England and Wales, and continue to increase their share of the dental market.

Career Highlight: Developing an innovative technique producing hollow prosthetic eyes

Emma Worrell

Workforce and workforce planning

Workforce planning is about 'ensuring the right numbers of people with the right skills are in the right place at the right time to provide the right services to the right people' (National Leadership and Innovation Agency for Healthcare, 2012).

I do not intend to include an analysis of dental workforce planning in the United Kingdom. That would be a book in itself. However, it is important to make reference to workforce planning because it will impact significantly on the working lives of all those currently working within dentistry and those planning to work in dentistry in the short to medium term.

It is important to match our workforce to the needs of the population. We need to match appropriate numbers and skills of dental professionals with the needs of our patients. Systems of dental care delivery have largely been built around the professionals giving the care rather than the people receiving it; that is, the patients. This is particularly true for those who are difficult to reach or easy to ignore: the homeless, sex workers, gypsies and travellers, people with physical or learning disabilities. As we move into the future, the dental profession will need to be more creative in how it addresses the oral health needs of its patients, particularly those just mentioned. In addition, the make-up of the dental workforce is likely to undergo a reshaping, with changes in the numbers and responsibilities of individual professional groups.

The Centre for Workforce Intelligence (2013) forecasts that by 2040 there will be an excess of between 1000 and 4000 dentists in the United Kingdom. Numbers for other dental professionals are not available. An excess of dentists will have an impact on future work prospects. The more dentists there are, the less work there will be for each dentist. Add to this the changing oral health needs of our patients, as I outline in Chapter 2, and it becomes obvious that the United Kingdom is likely to need fewer dentists, rather than more. However, it is also likely that the numbers of other dental professionals, such as dental hygienists and dental therapists, will rise. Direct access to some groups of DCPs will also have an impact. These factors and others will underpin a change in the profile of the profession, with fewer dentists and more DCPs. This transition, while an understandable reaction to the needs of the public and patients, will not be accomplished without difficulty. Increased clinical opportunities for some will be partnered by decreased clinical opportunities for others. This change is already underway – the 2013 report of the Centre for Workforce Intelligence reports that:

> Since 2008, there has been a steady shift in the make-up of the practice team. In 2008, dentists were 39 per cent of the dental team, but this proportion had dropped to 37 per cent by 2013. There has been an expansion in the numbers of dental nurses, dental technicians and orthodontic therapists, and the dental practice skill mix should change to reflect this.

Reviews of the dental workforce have also been undertaken in Scotland (Scottish Government, 2010), Wales (National Leadership and Innovation Agency for Healthcare, 2012) and Northern Ireland (Department of Health, Social Services and Public Safety in Northern Ireland, 2014). All of the workforce review reports make for interesting reading, and I would recommend looking at them as they can provide useful information for longer-term career planning.

> **Top Tip:** *Differentiate yourself – what is your unique selling point?*
>
> Reena Patel

Dentistry is a physical occupation. It takes its toll on our musculoskeletal system, our eyesight and our hearing. With age, manual dexterity can reduce. Add to that the psychological stress some in the profession suffer and it's easy to see why 30–40 years of clinical work is likely to prove problematic. I will consider the health of dental professionals in more detail in Chapter 2. It's another point in favour of the portfolio career. The majority of dental professionals will begin their careers with full-time clinical practice, which is a good way of honing your clinical skills and the craft of dentistry. It gives a solid foundation to the future. It's up to you how long that phase of your career lasts. Some people gain the skills and confidence to expand and diversify quicker than others. Some find the fulfilment of clinical practice is sufficient for many years. A few never lose the personal satisfaction of caring for their patients. Even to such dental professionals I would say, add some new experiences as you work through the years: flexibility and diversification are good for patients as well as for yourself. The dental professional who is constantly learning and who stays open to fresh ideas is likely to provide better patient care than the one who keeps their head down.

When thinking about building the shape of your working life, it may help to think about your personal and professional identity. Who are you? What is important to you? What is of little consequence? What do you definitely not want?

If you think I'm only appealing to dentists then I'd like to make it clear (again) that I think these opportunities are available to all who work in dentistry. The future, in my opinion, is very bright for non-dentist registrants.

If you think of a career as a palette of colours, what colour will your career be? A single block or a dazzling rainbow? Be the rainbow.

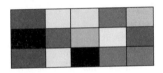

Top Tip: *Speak early in a meeting, this will give you confidence*
                                                                Janet Clarke

If you're lucky enough to do well, it's your responsibility to send the elevator back down

                                                                Kevin Spacey

I love this quote – keep sending those elevators (lifts, as we say in the United Kingdom) down.

Bibliography

Becker, M.J. (1999). Etrusan gold dental appliances: three newly 'discovered' examples. *Americal Journal of Archaeology*, **103**(1999), 103–111.

Bishop, M. (2014). 'Dentists' and the establishment of the Anglo-American dental profession in the eighteenth century: Part 1. The need for a name and an identity. *British Dental Journal*, **217**, 537–540.

British Association of Dental Therapists. History of the dental therapist. Available from: http://www.badt.org.uk/public/history-dental-therapist.html (last accessed 18 March 2015).

British Dental Association. (2013) *Business Trends Survey 2013: Findings from a Survey of UK Dentists*. London: BDA.

British Orthodontic Society. (2011). A history of the events which lead to the establishment of orthodontic therapists in the UK. http://www.bos.org.uk/Portals/0/Public/docs/Careers/History-of-Orthodontic-Therapists-2011.pdf (last accessed 18 March 2015).

Brousseau, K.R. and Driver, M.J (1994). Enhancing informed choice. A career concepts approach to career advancement. *The Magazine of the Graduate Management Admission Council*, **Spring**, 24 – 31.

Centre for Workforce Intelligence. (2013). A strategic review of the future dentistry workforce: informing dental student intake. Available from: http://www.cfwi.org.uk/publications/a-strategic-review-of-the-future-dentistry-workforce-informing-dental-student-intakes/ (last accessed 18 March 2015).

Dental Board of the UK. (1957). Minutes of the Dental Board of the UK for the Year 1956. Spottiswoode: Ballantyne & Co. Ltd.

Department of Health, Social Services and Public Safety in Northern Ireland. (2014). 2013/14 pay round. Available from: http://www.dhsspsni.gov.uk/sub_1037_2012_information_for_ddrb_2013_14.docx (last accessed 18 March 2015).

Dewey, J. (1916). *Democracy and Education: An Introduction to the Philosophy of Education*. Macmillian: London.

House of Commons Health Committee. (2006). NHS Charges. 3rd Report of Session 2005 – 06, Volume **1**, p.10.

National Leadership and Innovation Agency for Healthcare. (2012). An analysis of the dental workforce in Wales. Available from: http://www.weds.wales.nhs.uk/sitesplus/documents/1076/Analysis%20of%20Dental%20Workforce%20Wales%202012%20Full%20Report.pdf (last accessed 18 March 2015).

International Federation of Denturists. (2013). Available from: https://international-denturists.org/index.php/en/denturists-worldwide/denturism-an-overview (last accessed 18 March 2015).

Ipsos Mori. (2013). The NHS at 65. Available from: https://www.ipsos-mori.com/news events/blogs/makingsenseofsociety/1420/The-NHS-at-65.aspx (last accessed 18 March 2015).

Oxford University Press. (1996). *Oxford English Reference Dictionary*. Oxford University Press: Oxford, New York.

Royal College of Dental Surgeons of Ontario. (1899). *The Dental Advertiser*, Vol XX. Buffalo Dental Manufacturing Company: Buffalo, NY. Available from: http://booksnow1.scholarsportal.info/ebooks/oca7/53/dentaladvertise20buff/dental advertise20buff_bw.pdf (last accessed 18 March 2015).

Savickas, M.L., Nota, L., Rossier, J., *et al.* (2009) Life designing: a paradigm for career construction in the 21st century. *Journal of Vocational Behaviour*, 75, 239–250.

Scottish Government. (2010). An analysis of the dental workforce in Scotland: a strategic review. Available from: http://www.gov.scot/Publications/2011/03/07154848/21 (last accessed 18 March 2015).

Super, D.E., Savickas, M.L. and Super, C.M. (1996). The life-span, life-space approach to careers. In: Brown, D. and Brooks, L. (eds). *Career Choice and Development*, 3rd edn. Jossey-Bass: San Francisco, CA, pp. 121–178.

Chapter 2 Demography and society in the United Kingdom

```
        A               O
        G       S       R       T
    D   E   M   O   G   R   A   P   H   Y
                C           L       E       H
        K       I   N              E            E
        I       E                               A
    U   N   I   T   E   D                        L
        G       Y       M   A   R   K   E   T
        D               F                        H
    W   O   R   K       T   E   E   T   H
        M
```

> **Top Tip:** *Do as many different things as you can*
>
> Janine Brooks

As dental professionals we work in service to our patients. We work for society and as part of society. In this chapter, I want to consider how UK society is changing, particularly in the three major aspects of demography, working patterns and retirement. I wish to look at the general population and dental professionals and how changes to the general population affect the careers and working patterns of dental professionals. Why is this important? Dental professionals make their living in providing services to people; as those people change, there is an impact on dentistry and on provision of dental care and treatment. Our patients are how we make our livelihood; if we ignore changes in society then we may find our career travelling down a cul-de-sac. Understanding demography can also help when making career choices. People (patients) are our marketplace; it would be foolish to ignore market changes. In this chapter I will look at the demography of the general population of the United Kingdom and the demography of dental professionals. This will include the general health and oral health of the population. I will consider the health of dental professionals, working patterns in society and changing perceptions of retirement.

How to Develop Your Career in Dentistry, First Edition. Janine Brooks.
© 2015 John Wiley & Sons, Ltd. Published 2015 by John Wiley & Sons, Ltd.

Demography – general

Society, as we know, is changing. As a nation, we are getting older and can expect to live longer. The proportion of the population that is 65+ years is increasing: by 2032, the Office for National Statistics (2012) predicts those over the age of 65 will account for 22% of the total population, up from 18% in 2012 (Figure 2.1). Living longer is good news for us as individuals, but it may not be all good news for the whole of society, and it may not be good news for those who develop very poor health and live with that poor health for many years.

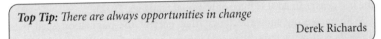

Top Tip: *There are always opportunities in change*

Derek Richards

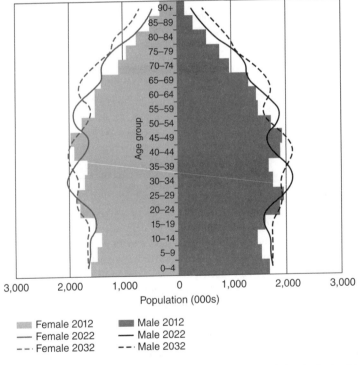

Figure 2.1 Projected change in the age structure of the population in England to 2032. Source: Office for National Statistics (2010). Statistical Bulletin. 2008-based subnational population projections. Reproduced with permission under the Open Government Licence: http://www.nationalarchives.gov.uk/doc/open-government-licence/version/2/ (last accessed 18 March 2015).

Population size

Figures 2.2 and 2.3 show the population growth in England between 1971 and 2011. Between 2012 and 2032 the population is predicted to grow by a further 8 million, to just over 61 million; this includes natural growth and net migration (Office for National Statistics, 2012).

The youngest age group, those under 20 years, is the only sector of the population that did not increase between 1971 and 2011. However, the National Census 2011 has shown that across England and Wales there was an increase of 13% in those aged under 5 years, with an increase of 6% in Scotland. Northern Ireland did not show an increase in this age group in the 10 years since the last census in 2001 (Office of National Statistics, 2012).

With increasing life expectancy, that part of the population aged over 65 years is growing faster than that under 65 years of age. Between 2012 and 2032, those aged between 65 and 84 years will rise by 39%, and those over 85 years by 106%.

An interesting metric is the old-age dependency ratio, or the number of people of pension age and over for every 1000 people of working age. With current pension ages, the ratio is predicted to be 375 in 2021, rising to 492 in 2051. Even with the planned changes to pension age, the ratio is predicted to be 358 in 2041 and 342 in 2051 (Office for National Statistics, 2012). This also means that there will be fewer people working to pay for the pensions of those who are retired.

> *Top Tip: Don't be afraid to say you are wrong and apologise*
>
> Janet Clarke

Population age

The King's Fund (2012) has published work demonstrating that, since 1981, average life expectancy has increased from 71 to 79 years for men and from 77 to 87 years for women: a massive 9 and 10 years of extra life expectancy in only 30 years. By 2032, it is expected to increase to 83 and 87 years, respectively.

In 1901, baby boys were expected to live for 45 years and girls for 49 years. Of babies born in 2014, one-third can expect to reach their 100th birthday; this rises to 40% for girls.

Medical advances, future patterns of disease and population behaviour could all have a significant impact on life expectancy, driving it either up or down.

> *Career Highlight: Working full time while bringing up two children*
>
> Janet Clarke

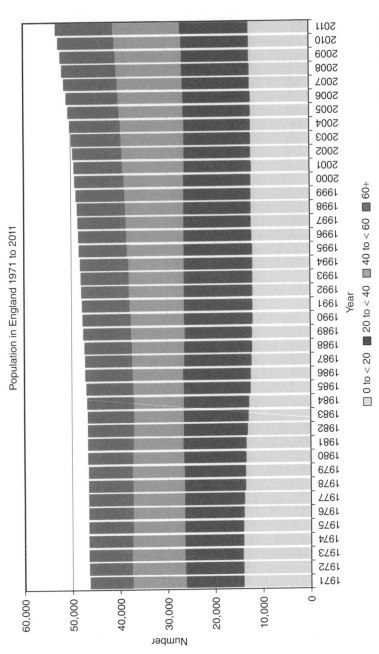

Figure 2.2 Population in England, 1971–2011. Source: ONS mid-year population estimates, NHAIS. Reproduced with permission under the Open Government Licence: http://www.nationalarchives.gov.uk/doc/open-government-licence/version/2/ (last accessed 18 March 2015).

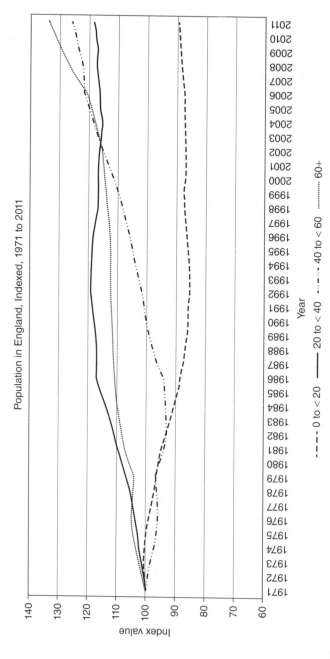

Figure 2.3 Population in England, indexed, 1971–2011. Source: ONS mid-year population estimates, NHAIS. Reproduced with permission under the Open Government Licence: http://www.nationalarchives.gov.uk/doc/open-government-licence/version/2/ (last accessed 18 March 2015).

General health

Healthy life expectancy is growing at a similar rate to general life expectancy, suggesting that the extra years of life will not necessarily be years of ill health. So, we are living healthier, longer lives. This is good news, but there will of course be consequences to more of us living longer. In this book I'm concerned about the dental implications, and in particular how they will impact on the career choices of dental professionals. I will not attempt to predict the exact impact, but I hope I can shine a light on those aspects of demography that dental professionals choosing career opportunities might want to take into consideration. More of that later, once the scene has been set.

From a general health point of view, older age can bring difficulties. The number of people with some disease will double over the next 20 years. The King's Fund (2012) states that the number of people in England with three or more long-term conditions is expected to rise from 1.9 million in 2008 to 2.9 million in 2018 (Figure 2.4). By 2018, it is estimated that there will be 7 million older people who cannot walk up a flight of stairs without resting and 1 million people aged 75+ who find it difficult to get to their local hospital. By 2025, cases of diabetes, particularly type II, are predicted to rise by 29% to 4 million. By 2030, there will be 17 million people with arthritis and over

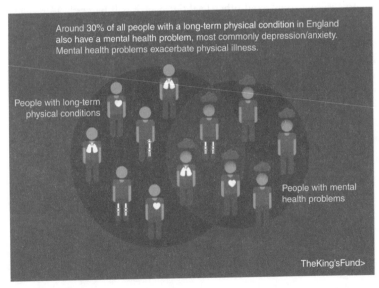

Figure 2.4 Proportion of the population with physical and mental health problems (England) 2012. Source: The King's Fund. Time to Think Differently. http://www.kingsfund.org.uk/time-to-think-differently/audio-video/case-change-slide-pack. Last accessed 18 March 2015. Reproduced with permission of The King's Fund.

3 million living with cancer. Further, by 2030, the number of older people with care needs is predicted to rise by 61%. Old age can trigger a number of debilitating conditions, including sight and hearing loss and dementia. The number living with dementia are expected to rise to 1.4 million by 2042. The number of cases of infection with human immunodeficiency virus (HIV) are continuing to rise. Antimicrobial-resistant bacteria could undermine the effectiveness of some medicines.

Long-term conditions are more prevalent in older people: 58% of people over the age of 60 years, compared to 14% of those under 40. People in the poorest social class have a 60% higher prevalence than those in the richest social class, and 30% greater severity of disease.

The prevalence of obesity has risen from 15% in 1993 to 26% in 2010 (Figure 2.5) (The Health and Social Care Information Centre, 2011). Some predictions suggest that by 2035, 46% of men and 40% of women will be obese, resulting in more than 550 000 cases of diabetes and around 400 000 additional cases of heart disease and stroke (Wang *et al.*, 2011).

The predicted increase in people with obesity has serious implications for dental services from the point of view of both the systemic disease it is associated with and the provision and management of dental care for the obese individual. For example, there will be an increased need for specialist dental chairs, waiting rooms and other facilities, which will be costly to provide.

More than **6 out of 10 men** are overweight or obese

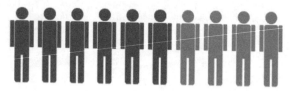

More than **5 out of 10 women** are overweight or obese

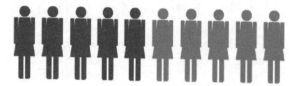

Figure 2.5 Proportion of males and females overweight or obese, 2010. Source: The King's Fund. Time to Think Differently. http://www.kingsfund.org.uk/time-to-think -differently/audio-video/case-change-slide-pack. Last accessed 18 March 2015. Reproduced with permission of The King's Fund.

Post-weight-loss surgery can affect the oral tissues. There are pharmacological considerations, too. Bariatric dentistry will become an increasingly well known aspect of dental care.

More positively, smoking rates have fallen to around 20%, but the rate of decline is slow at 0.4% per year. Smoking is one of the primary reasons for the gap in life expectancy between rich and poor (The Health and Social Care Information Centre, 2011).

> **Top Tip:** *Plan and organise your day*
>
> Emma Worrell

The past century has seen a shift from communicable diseases, such as tuberculosis and typhoid, to noncommunicable diseases, such as cancer and heart disease. This, alongside the continued decline in mortality rates and growing life expectancy, means that disease, in the main, is something that people now live with rather than die from (Barnett *et al.*, 2012).

Snell *et al.* (2011) estimate that the number of younger adults with learning disabilities will rise by over 32% between 2010 and 2030, from around 220 000 to about 290 000, and the number of younger adults with physical or sensory impairment by 7.5% over the same period, from under 3 million to just over 3 million.

Another important trend is the increasing number of alcohol-related deaths from liver disease. In 2012, there were 8367 alcohol-related deaths in the United Kingdom. In the last 30 years, mortality has risen by over 450% in this country (Academy of Medical Sciences, 2009).

The King's Fund (2012) report urges us to think differently about health and social care. These changes will have a considerable impact on dentistry and on dental professionals providing a service. The impact on our career choices also needs to be considered carefully. These data and predictions point to an increasing need for dental professionals to acquire skills in geriodontology and special needs dentistry.

> **Career Highlight:** *Being selected as a GDC Educational Inspector*
>
> Shazad Malik

Oral health

The oral health of the UK population is improving for most dental diseases, in some areas dramatically, in others more slowly. Oral health adult surveys have shown an excellent and impressive improvement in the retention of natural teeth in the older sectors of the population. Surveys of adult oral health have been carried out every 10 years since 1968 in the United Kingdom; the fifth such survey was completed in 2009 in England, Wales and Northern Ireland (Scotland did not take part in the 2009 survey). These surveys provide a valuable window on trends in the oral health of our patients and are an important factor to consider in our careers.

The drop in people who have lost all their teeth is particularly impressive. In 1968, 36% of the adult population was edentulous; by the Adult Dental Health Survey of 2009, this had fallen to about 8%: a truly dramatic decrease (Figure 2.6). In England, Wales and Northern Ireland, 94% of the combined population was dentate (defined as having at least one natural tooth). The majority of dentate adults (60%) had between 27 and 32 teeth. In a relatively few years, dentures, and certainly complete dentures, have become much less commonplace – even rare in some parts of the country.

For those under 45, the likelihood of retaining not just some teeth, but a considerable number of healthy teeth through the whole of a long life, is now very high. In particular, the prospects for young adults aged 16 to 24 look better than they have ever been [see Figure 2.7].

With retention of teeth comes dental caries. The 2009 Adult Dental Health Survey found that just under one-third of dentate adults (31%) had obvious tooth decay in either the crowns or the roots of their teeth. For those adults who had some decay, the average number of teeth affected was 2.7. There may be less need for complete dentures today, but restoration of teeth and partial dentures still needs to be provided.

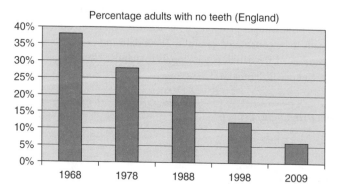

Figure 2.6 Percentage of adults in England with no teeth, 1968–2009. Source: Adult Dental Health Survey.

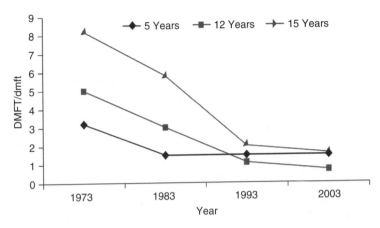

Figure 2.7 Changes in mean dmft/DMFT for children in the United Kingdom, 1973–2003. Source: http://webarchive.nationalarchives.gov.uk/20130107105354/ http://www.dh.gov.uk/prod_consum_dh/groups/dh_digitalassets/@dh/@en /documents/digitalasset/dh_4123885.pdf (last accessed 18 March 2015). Reproduced with permission under the Open Government Licence: http://webarchive .nationalarchives.gov.uk/20130107105354/http://www.nationalarchives.gov.uk/doc /open-government-licence/open-government-licence.htm.(last accessed 18 March 2015).

> **Top Tip:** *Demonstrate reliability*
>
> Debbie White

Other oral conditions seem to be on the increase; for example, while severe tooth wear remains rare, there are signs of an increase between the adult dental health surveys of 1999 and 2009. There is a small but increasing proportion of younger adults with moderate wear that is likely to be clinically important.

An interesting paper by Wieder *et al.* (2013) calls into question the ability of dental schools to teach dental students the skills of providing complete dentures. In their conclusion, Wieder *et al.* write:

> *Competence in complete dentures falls short of what is expected. With a single exception all the schools seem to have low expectations for their undergraduate students to be practically trained and experienced in the production of complete dentures.*

Could the skills for provision of complete dentures be moving from the undergraduate to the postgraduate domain?

> **Top Tip:** *Be professional*
>
> Bal Chana

In 40 years, the proportion of 5-year-old children in England with no experience of dental caries has risen from just under 30% to just over 70%, a massive reduction in disease level (Figure 2.8). However, there is still variation across the country, with the South East showing the lowest level of caries and the North West the highest. This is important information when considering where to work. Figure 2.9 shows the variation with 95% confidence limits for the different regions of England.

> **Career Highlight:** *Obtaining a Specialty post in Dental Public Health*
>
> Reena Patel

Unlike dental caries levels, which are generally falling, periodontal disease levels are not. In the Adult Dental Health Survey of 2009, 17% of dentate adults were shown to have very healthy periodontal tissues, with no periodontal disease; that is, no bleeding, no calculus, no periodontal pockets of

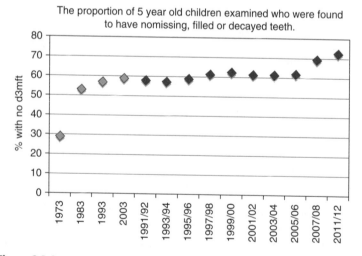

Figure 2.8 Proportion of 5-year-old children with no missing, filled or decayed teeth, 1973–2011/12. Source: Data are taken from results of caries surveys of five-year-olds in England from the Children's Dental Health Surveys and NHS Dental Epidemiology surveys, 1973 to 2012. http://www.nwph.net/dentalhealth/Oral%20Health%205yr%20old%20children%202012%20final%20report%20gateway%20approved.pdf (last accessed 18 March 2015).

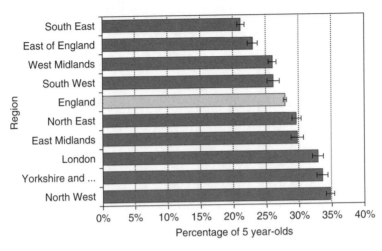

Figure 2.9 Variation in proportion of 5-year-old children in England with experience of dental caries, with 95% confidence limits, 2011/12. Source: Data are taken from results of caries surveys of five-year-olds in England from the Children's Dental Health Surveys and NHS Dental Epidemiology surveys, 1973 to 2012. http://www.nwph.net /dentalhealth/Oral%20Health%205yr%20old%20children%202012%20final%20 report%20gateway%20approved.pdf (last accessed 18 March 2015).

>4 mm (Figure 2.10). Among dentate adults, 10% showed excellent oral health. The proportion of the population with healthy periodontal tissues and no calculus or bleeding on probing was highest in 16–24 year olds, at 28%, but fell to 10% among those over the age of 85 years. This should not be surprising when one considers that the population is retaining teeth for longer. The population is also living longer, and more teeth for more years of life means more periodontal tissues exposed to the likelihood of disease.

> **Top Tip:** *Be positive, anything is possible*
>
> Sophie Noske

The series of graphs in Figure 2.11 demonstrates the trend for the population to retain more and healthier teeth even into late older age.

The burden of oral disease is changing. As time progresses, there will be more mild or moderate disease and less severe disease. There is likely to be less need for interventions, but, when required, interventions will be more complex. There is probably a scale of disease between mild/moderate and severe, with not much in the middle.

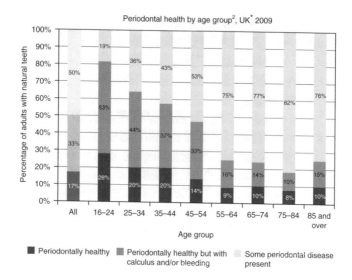

Figure 2.10 Periodontal health by age group in the United Kingdom, 2009. Source: Adult Dental Health Survey.

You may be thinking, why have I included all this interesting 'stuff' on the demographics of society and patients? This is supposed to be a book about developing careers in dentistry. The reason is that the future dental workforce and our future career patterns need to be firmly based on future work. We are a service industry that only exists because patients need us. We must match use of this knowledge in planning and extending our careers or we may find ourselves up a dental blind alley.

Most of the dental professionals who will be working in 20 years' time are already working in dentistry today, so this book is as much, if not more, for those who are already within the profession than those registrants just starting out. The information contained in these pages will help you as you think about profiling and reprofiling your career over the years.

> **Top Tip:** *Always have time for your family*
>
> Sophie Noske

A greater number of older people in the population will lead to a greater number of people with more complex health needs and complicated medical histories: polypharmacy, for example. These patients will present challenges in their dental treatment and management. It is likely there will be an increased need for dental professionals skilled in special care dentistry.

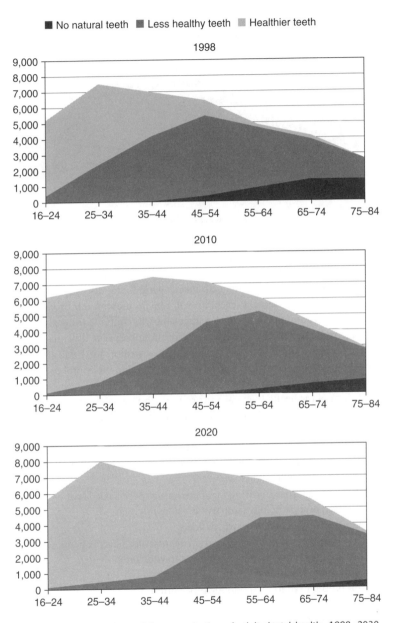

Figure 2.11 Time series and future projection of adult dental health, 1998–2030. 'Healthier' is defined as having 18 or more sound, untreated teeth. 'Less healthy' is defined as having less than 18 sound, untreated teeth. Source: Improving Dental Care & Oral Health – A call to action evidence resource pack, NHS England, Feb. 14 Gateway ref: 01173. Data taken from the Adult Dental Health Surveys 1998 & 2009, Health and Social Information Centre. http://www.england.nhs.uk/ourwork/qual-clin-lead/calltoaction/dental-call-to-action/ http://www.england.nhs.uk/wp-content/uploads/2014/04/cta-dent-evid-pack.pdf (last accessed 18 March 2015).

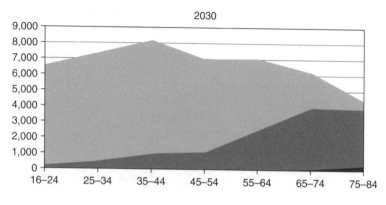

Figure 2.11 *(continued)*

More older people with more teeth is likely to lead to an increase in advanced restorative treatment needs, as people remain keen to keep their ageing dentition. Of course, more natural teeth means periodontal disease will remain an important oral disease. Prevention will remain high on our professional agenda. Xerostomia is unlikely to reduce and will continue to need careful management. This will have implications for the appropriate skill mix among dental professionals. Thus, more older patients with more teeth will affect the career choices of dental professionals. Oral cancer and other oral pathology conditions are also likely to be an increasing health issue.

Looking at the health (general and oral), age and size of the population can help us reach some conclusions and predictions for oral needs in the future. My predictions are:

- Increased expertise in caring for and treating older people.
- Increased expertise in complex restoration of the older dentition.
- Increased periodontal disease.
- Increased expertise in caring for and treating special-needs patient.
- Increased oral pathology (soft-tissue lesions).
- Increased numbers of bariatric patients.
- Possible increased numbers of partial dentures for older patients.
- Less need for implants (fewer teeth lost to younger patients).
- Continuing demand for cosmetic procedures.
- Continuing need for orthodontic procedures.

Health of dentists

There are few data on the health of the dental profession, and the majority of what does exist is about dentists rather than all registrant groups. However, the important message from what is available is that dentistry is a demanding profession, physically, mentally and emotionally, for all those who work in it. It is useful to place this statement in the context of research that has been undertaken into the health of dental practitioners working in the UK. Ailments concerning the locomotor apparatus, cardiovascular problems and neurotic symptoms have been identified as the main causes of British dentists leaving the profession before normal retirement age (Burke *et al.*, 1997).

The prevalence of musculoskeletal complaints in dentists is high and has been demonstrated in a wide variety of self-reported questionnaire-based studies. Types of problem include back pain and neck, shoulder and hand/wrist complaints. Research shows that the physical nature of dental clinical work seems to place dentists at risk of developing musculoskeletal disorders. A survey by Kay and Scarrott (1997) found that 22% of British dentists experienced so much physical pain that it had limiting effects on their ability to work as a dentist, possibly compromising clinical performance.

> **Top Tip:** *Address things that scare you*
>
> Reena Patel

It is generally accepted that dentists encounter numerous sources of stress throughout their careers, beginning as early as when they are at dental school (Newbury-Birch *et al.*, 2002). On entering general dental practice, the number and variety of organisational and individual stressors can often grow (Kay and Lowe, 2008). For some dentists, these issues may significantly affect their general and/or mental health (Myers and Myers, 2004). Clinical disorders such as burnout (Gorter *et al.*, 1998) and depression (Gale, 1998) may then result.

Myers and Myers (2004) investigated overall stress, work stress and health in general dental practitioners. A comparatively large number of dentists reported high levels of psychological stress symptoms, such as being nervy, tense and depressed; some even showed minor psychiatric symptoms; 58% reported headaches, 60% reported difficulty in sleeping and 48% reported feeling tired for no apparent reason. These were all related to work stress.

The literature demonstrates how many dentists develop stress disorders early in their careers, and studies have shown increasing evidence of stress-related problems in young dentists and dental students (Humphris, 1999; Newbury-Birch *et al.*, 2002; Willet and Palmer, 2009).

Gilmour *et al.* (2005) undertook research to assess career satisfaction among a group of general dental practitioners in Staffordshire. Their objectives were to assess the level of job satisfaction among general dental practitioners from one area of England and to assess the association of various personal and work-related factors with job satisfaction. Their conclusions were that:

> Overall, job satisfaction showed a high correlation with overall professional satisfaction, delivery of care, income, respect and professional time. Significantly higher job satisfaction scores were identified amongst dentists with a special area of interest, those practising privately, and in non-rural locations.

I was particularly interested by the conclusion that job satisfaction showed a high correlation with those with a special area of interest. It would be fascinating to see the effect of portfolio careers on the overall satisfaction of dental professionals. I suggest that those who have a diverse career are more likely to have higher levels of job satisfaction (and personal satisfaction) than those who do not. Will this protect against health problems? It would be nice to think so, but there is no evidence as yet from which to draw conclusions. However, it seems sensible to suggest that a combination of clinical and non-clinical work might reduce the physical ailments that dental professionals are prone to develop and might also reduce psychological stress.

> *A dream doesn't become reality through magic; it takes sweat, determination and hard work*
>
> Colin Powell

Dental care professionals

The future opportunities for DCP registrants are, in my opinion, very bright, with a number of ways to develop. The demographics of the patient base in the United Kingdom points towards a greater emphasis on prevention. As people live longer and keep their teeth into a ripe old age, periodontal disease will become even more important. It seems likely that dentists will develop specialist skills while more routine dental treatments become the province of dental therapists, dental hygienists and dental nurses. Direct access will become a driver, but it isn't the only factor: patient demographics will also play a role. Dentistry and the dental profession are entering a period of radical change, one not seen since the inception of the NHS.

> **Top Tip:** *Sleep on tricky decisions*
>
> Janet Clarke

Working patterns

We know that society is changing constantly. In this section, I will be considering societal change from the point of view of the length of our working lives. What people want from the jobs they do also seems to be changing. The New Career Paradigm, an interesting piece of work undertaken by David Blustein (2006), suggests that people make decisions about the work they want to do based on work/life balance, opportunities to learn and grow and benefits, as well as how well a job pays. Blustein brought a relational approach to careers. This builds on the work of Super *et al.* (1996) outlined in Chapter 1. The research undertaken in North America showed that people moved jobs five to six times during their working lives and made two to three major career changes. It seems that people now want much more from their work – more than their parents or grandparents did. They want to tailor their careers to their individual requirements, rather than just expecting to follow well-trodden traditional career paths. In addition, those individual requirements often change as they travel through their lives and careers.

Those under 30 years of age

In dentistry, members of this group are usually up to seven years post-qualification. They are keen, enthusiastic and committed to their profession. They want meaningful work and a good work/home balance. At this stage, salary is important; there are probably university fees to repay, substantial professional costs and high living expenses.

Those in their 30s

These professionals have several years of work experience, feel confident in their abilities and may be taking further qualifications. They are taking on more responsibilities, but they may also feel frustrated and dissatisfied if their career is not progressing as they thought it would: the 'same old, same old' syndrome. They are looking for challenge and development. At the same time, they may have family commitments and young children, and may be taking career breaks. This can be a stressful decade.

Those in their 40s

These professionals are highly experienced and skilled, may be specialising in aspects of dentistry, are growing and ready for more. However, this can be when job satisfaction begins to wane. Children are growing up but are still demanding of their parents as they enter late teens and university. This is a good decade to capitalise on experience and grow the portfolio.

Those in their 50s

Job benefits become key for many in this decade. Health issues may emerge and older parents can become a concern just as children have flown the nest for good (although, for some, this may take a while). There can be dissatisfaction that their talents are not used more. However, this can be a prime time to use their years of experience and diversify. Those who have taken career breaks or worked part time for a while may be looking for more from their jobs. This can be the time to take on more opportunities outside the surgery if they couldn't earlier.

Those in their 60s and beyond

This is a great time to diversify, and flexible work options are again a driver at this point in their career. These professionals have so much to offer and are eager to offer it. Clinical work may feel physically and mentally much more demanding, and now is the time to really benefit from all that networking and to work the portfolio, expanding nonclinical roles.

Career Highlight: Pioneering direct access for dental therapists

Bal Chana

Impact on dental professionals

> *Patient and public expectations are rising. Increasingly, patients and service users expect health and social care services to be like other service industries and are willing to do more for themselves and interact with services via technology. They expect to be offered choice and variety and to experience services that are convenient, personalised and provided in modern buildings and healing environments*

> King's Fund (2012)

As providers of a service to the public, we need to respond positively to the public's expectations: we ignore them at our peril. It is encouraging that the King's Fund quote suggests that patients are willing to do more for themselves; this bodes well for a truly meaningful partnership between dentist and patient.

In the retail world, availability 7 days of the week is the norm and is expected. I can remember a time when it was impossible to do your weekly food shop on Sunday, because most shops were not open, but those times have long gone. Why then are we still so taken with the weekend? Why do we work to a pattern of 5 : 2, taking Saturday and Sunday off? Is this appropriate for today's society? Since I have become a sole trader, working for myself, the idea of not working on a Saturday or a Sunday seems odd. I work when I want to and take time off when I want to. Wednesday has become the new Saturday. It's rather nice taking time for me and the family in the week rather than when everyone else is manically trying to cram in their leisure time, at the weekend. Why not open your surgery until 8 pm three evenings a week and then have the rest of the time to do other things? Why not work Saturday and Sunday and then take 2 days off during the week? A day is just 24 hours, regardless of the name we give those 24 hours. We are becoming more creative in how we use our time and I think we will become still more so in the future. In my book, there is no such thing as work/life balance: it's just balance. Each of us needs to work out our own balance and the balance you choose will be unique to you. With a portfolio career, balance is the key. So, provided you still find work stimulating and your health is up to it, I suggest retirement is an outmoded concept in need of redefinition.

Changes to the demography of our patient base will be supplemented by changes for us as individuals and by changes in our working lives.

Is it sensible to expect dental professionals to continue working 5 days a week until they reach their 70s or even 80s? It may be for some, but not for all. Indeed, it seems an unrealistic expectation for all. Dentistry, as I outlined earlier, is a physical occupation, and the health issues alone could make such long working lives as practitioners providing direct patient care difficult. Dentistry puts strains on the vision, hearing, manual dexterity and musculoskeletal systems – not to mention the psychological strains. Individual professionals may be keen to retain some working commitment, but might find direct clinical care impossible. The good news is that dentistry offers satisfying and stretching intellectual options. The days of remaining on a single career track for your whole working life are probably gone, and in many ways that's not a bad thing.

> **Top Tip:** *No regrets, go for it*
>
> Sophie Noske

Working lives and patterns of working are changing, and are likely to continue to change radically.

I noted previously that patient and public expectations are rising, and it is unlikely that this trend will reverse. Patients expect more from their dental care: they want choice, they want to be involved in their care and they are not afraid to say what they want from dentistry and dental professionals.

Within dentistry and health care, we are fortunate that change is constant. Do you find that alarming? Change is stimulating: it brings fresh opportunities and challenge. Of course, there has been much research to show that individuals say they don't like change; we have an industry of change management. However, that same research reveals it isn't necessarily the change that people find difficult: it's whether or not they are in control of it (Lewin, 1947). If we are (or feel we are) in control of change then we can relish it. Dental professionals are more likely to be in a position of control. If you don't think you are then you may feel more alarmed or unsettled by change, which you perceive to be imposed. A portfolio career could be proof against finding change a challenge: if one part of your portfolio changes out of your control, other aspects may not. Plus, you make the change.

> **Top Tip:** *Be kind to yourself – we can be our hardest critics*
>
> Emma Worrell

Technology rising

Technological advances in genetics, biotechnology, material sciences and bioinformatics are fast and furious. Low-cost genetic sequencing, genome mapping, biomarker tests and targeted drugs and treatments could enable professionals to provide tailored health information and create personalised treatments to improve patient outcomes (Cho *et al.*, 2014). These are all growing fields and will all revolutionise health care in the future, including dentistry, either directly or indirectly.

There is increasing impetus to deliver care through video conferencing supported by the digital transfer of clinical information. This could include remote intensive-care monitoring systems. Robotics-based surgical procedures are also growing rapidly (Barbash and Glied, 2010). It is likely that these techniques will revolutionise the accuracy with which dentistry can be performed, conserving far more healthy tissue.

New technologies and models of care, workforce trends and changing skill mixes are all factors for change, but it is not certain exactly what their impact will be.

Demand for highly skilled individuals is growing, while automation threatens the jobs of the less skilled. Information technology is blurring the boundaries between work and home, facilitating part-time and remote working. Changes to pension provision mean that people can expect to work for longer.

> **Top Tip:** *Never look down on anyone, always be grateful*
>
> Shazad Malik

The King's Fund (2012) tells us:

Current models of care also appear to be outmoded at a time when society and technologies are evolving rapidly and are changing the way in which we interact with each other and with service providers. While health and social care services have evolved since the establishment of the NHS, change has been much slower than in other industries such as banking and retailing, where the use of technology has transformed the relationship between service providers and their customers. Experience in other countries where health care organisations have already embraced new technologies indicates the shape of things to come and the potential to deliver care more effectively.

We are seeing the change in how dentistry is delivered. Our relationship with our patients is much more of a partnership than it was years ago.

Top Tip: *Take opportunities when they arise*

Debbie White

The demands of dental practice are well documented. Accordingly, one would ordinarily expect that most dentists would not work until their 70s before retiring from clinical practice. Table 2.1 shows the number of dentists

Table 2.1 Age of dentists registered with General Dental Council (31 March 2013)

Age/number	Total	Proportion
All dentists	40 420	100%
20–24	1018	2.5%
25–29	5774	14%
30–34	5907	15%
35–39	6041	15%
40–44	4972	12%
45–49	4758	12%
50–54	4563	11%
55–59	3728	9%
60–64	2093	5%
65+	1551	4%
Unknown	15	0.03%

Note: The proportions have been rounded up and therefore exceed 100%.
Source: General Dental Council.

currently registered with the General Dental Council by age group. With a peak at 30–39 years (30% of dentists), the population is relatively steady until 55 years of age, when it begins to reduce. The data show that there are 7372 registered dentists aged 55+ years (18% of the total). Until now, most dentists have been able to make healthy provision for their retirement through pensions – but for well known reasons, that is now changing for all self-employed and many employed individuals. There are plainly no data for the future, but what is clear is that, like the rest of the population, dentists now will have to work for more years than they have done in the past.

> **Career Highlight**: *Completing a MDPH during maternity leave*
>   Reena Patel

Table 2.2 breaks down all DCPs registered with the GDC at 31 March 2013 by age and professional group. The remarkable fact I discovered when analysing these data is that a large number of DCPs are registered in more than one professional category. I have only counted each person once, but there are many professionals registered in two, three and four categories. I feel this demonstrates professional drive and that dentistry is a profession in which those with the will and capability can build a career unique to themselves.

I have highlighted the largest age group in each profession. Dental nurses are a particularly young group, showing an age peak of 25–29 years. Hygienists, technicians and clinical dental technicians all show an age

Table 2.2 DCPs registered with the General Dental Council, by age and professional group (31 March 2013)

Age	Total	Dental nurse	Therapist	Hygienist	Technician	Ortho therapist	Clinical DT
All	63 010	49 780	2213	4327	6098	323	269
20–24	6462	6114	177	28	133	10	
25–29	**17 826**	**10 170**	524	176	432	61	1
30–34	10 087	8371	**560**	430	622	**82**	21
35–39	8141	6366	328	583	765	65	34
40–44	7821	5963	219	729	817	51	42
45–49	6732	4767	108	**813**	**974**	27	**46**
50–54	5812	3939	121	745	949	15	43
55–59	4067	2711	121	497	685	11	42
60–64	1775	1060	45	234	407	1	28
65+	743	315	10	92	314		12
Not known	4	4					

Source: General Dental Council.

Table 2.3 Self-reported expected age at retirement, BDA members (2013)

Age	Yes	No	Don't know	Total number
<35	0.5%	99.0%	0.5%	209
35–44	1.5%	97.1%	1.5%	340
45–54	1.6%	96.2%	2.2%	445
55–64	21.4%	70.1%	8.5%	318
65+	29.7%	48.6%	21.6%	37
Total				**1349**

peak at 45–49 years. Dental therapists show a younger age peak at 30–34 years. Only 10% of all DCP professional groups taken as a whole are aged 55+ years.

Top Tip: Strive to be the best

Bal Chana

At present, dentists working in the NHS can take their pension from age 60 without financial penalty. This will eventually rise to 68, but how many dentists will want to continue working clinically to this age? If they do, will they wish to work full time?

In 2013, the BDA asked its members if they planned to retire in the next year. Table 2.3 shows the results. While the numbers responding to the survey are relatively low, the table does show an interesting feature: just under half of those practitioners aged over 65 years had no plans to retire.

Retirement

John F. Kennedy once said, 'Change is the law of life. And those who look only to the past or present are certain to miss the future.' This is certainly true of preparing for retirement. If we continue to expect that the ways of the past will see us through to our futures, we will be left behind. The methods that helped prepare us for retirement are quickly disappearing, and we must start using others. However, I would suggest that turning our attention now and then to the past or present can be beneficial in moulding our future. Of course, I'm nit-picking here as Kennedy does say those who look *only*.

In 1908, when Lloyd George introduced state pensions for those aged 70 years and above, the average person could expect about 9 years of retirement. In 2013, as a society, we are enjoying more years of retirement, while our years of work have reduced, as most people will have retired before the age of 70. The state is thus having to find more money to pay more pensioners for more years. This is reinforced by work carried out by the Organisation for Economic Co-operation and Development (OECD, 2013), which produced a report on retirement and pensions across a number of countries and reported that, in the United Kingdom, males could expect 19.1 years of retirement (average age at retirement 63.7 years), while females could expect 22.1 years of retirement (average age at retirement 63.2 years). It also seems that as people live longer, we have begun to retire earlier: a double economic whammy. Clearly, this has produced a serious economic issue. Pension age fell to 60 for women and 65 for men for many years, but this has reversed and state pension age is scheduled to rise to 67 years by 2034 and 68 years by 2046. So, what are the possible consequences of these changes? Clearly, both good and bad.

Roger Ramsden, chief executive of Saga Services, says: 'While some people delay retirement for financial reasons, we're finding an increasing number of people are staying in the workforce because they enjoy what they do, they like to keep their mind and body active and because they enjoy socialising with work colleagues' (Ramsden, 2013). OECD found that one in three people is working past what was their retirement age.

We know society is not what it used to be; certainly, retirement isn't. What do I mean? I mean that the concept of working one day and not working the next is changing. Many people keep an element of work for as many days in the week as they wish to. And why not? Why should dental professionals be any different?

Someone born in 1997 and entering dental training in 2015 can currently expect to receive a state pension in 2065 when they are 68 years of age. Of course, for a dental professional, the state pension may not be seen as the major impacting factor on when they decide to begin their retirement. Most will still have an occupational pension or private pension to look forward to. However, economics aside, working in a demanding profession such as dentistry may not retain its appeal when an individual is 65+ years old.

> **Top Tip:** *Develop your own leadership style*
>
> Reena Patel

Retirement as our parents understood it might soon cease to exist, if it hasn't already done so. As most of us enjoy good health and longer lives, finishing work at 60 or 65 years of age, or any specific age, is losing its relevance, and perhaps even its appeal. I've realised as I approach the traditional age to hang up my 'mirror and probe' that I'm not ready to, and I actually don't want to lose the buzz of working. Those who retain interests – and I include an interesting occupation here – are more likely to remain healthier, both physically and mentally, and probably live longer. Of course, there are also economic considerations for some. Not everyone will be able to afford to retire completely in the comparatively young decade of their 60s. The Baby Boomers have reached retirement with greater wealth and more generous pensions than any other generation before them – possibly ever. In 2014, the Baby Boomers were aged between 50 and 68 years. They will continue to use health services, and in particular dental services, for the next 30–50 years. Many will have the resources to pay for private health care and private dental care.

Economics must have an influence on our working patterns, including how long we work for and how much work we do. If our domestic commitments increase, our requirement for money will probably also increase. In the future, individuals are more likely to have several marriages or long-term partnerships; women are delaying starting their families or are having second, perhaps third families. So, children may still be at school or university when their parents might traditionally have thought about retirement. My suggestion is that dental professionals are less likely to be retiring fully in their mid 50s to 60s. However, I don't foresee that this means 5 days' clinical working for everyone. In fact, as dentistry is both a physically and mentally demanding profession, working full time in direct patient care is probably not possible or desirable. Studies suggest that dental professionals suffer musculoskeletal, sensory, cognitive and psychological detrimental effects as they get older, which makes demanding, precise surgical procedures more challenging. While it's not impossible to be a competent clinician into one's 80s, it seems rather aspirational to assume everyone will manage it. However, diversifying and developing a portfolio-type working pattern is most definitely a viable way forward; indeed, I would suggest it's the only way forward. Even for those professionals who utterly adore direct patient care, diversity keeps you fresh and enthusiastic for dentistry, and patients must clearly benefit from being treated by dental professionals who relish the work they do. A portfolio career is achievable by all dental professionals – and I do mean all, not just dentists. I've included case studies in Chapter 5 from across the profession; hopefully you will find them inspiring and informative.

A study undertaken by Stewart *et al.* (2007) looked at the career intentions, work/life balance and retirement plans of senior dental students. The study used self-reported questionnaires and included students from dental schools in Manchester and Dundee. There were 141 responses, equating to a response rate of 78%. The results highlight several points of interest. At that time, the majority of students intended to begin work in general dental practice (65%). The questionnaire asked at what age the students intended to retire or leave full-time dentistry: about a fifth planned to work

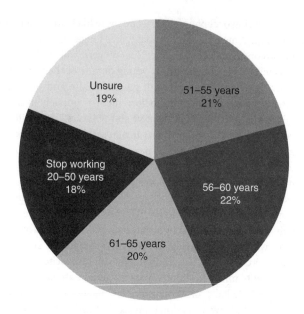

Figure 2.12 Self-reported expected age at retirement, Manchester and Dundee dental students (2007).

until they were 56–60 years, and another fifth planned to work until they were aged 61–65 years (Figure 2.12). What is even more interesting is that a further two-fifths reported that their intention was to stop working in dentistry before the age of 55 years, with 18% expressing their aspiration to retire from dentistry before they were 50. What did they anticipate doing post-dentistry? Full-time non-work? A different type of work? The study reported that the majority intended to work part time in dentistry following retirement from full-time dentistry. Just under a quarter of the male students stated they would work part time in another job, compared to only 2% of the female students; 3% of the male students and 6% of the females anticipated starting a different full-time career. Similar proportions of both sexes stated their intention to do no further paid work.

> **Top Tip:** *Map out your vision and career destination – it doesn't matter if you don't follow through!*
>
> Reena Patel

Since the paper by Stewart *et al.* (2007) was published, changes to the UK pension scheme have been announced. From 2020, everyone (men and women) will need to work until 65 years of age before receiving their state pension. It could be that a similar study undertaken now with senior students might produce different result.

> **Career Highlight:** *Member of Mount Abu Cleft Team*
>
> Emma Worrell

Bibliography

Academy of Medical Sciences. (2009). Calling time: the nation's drinking as a major health issue. Available from: http://www.acmedsci.ac.uk/policy/policy/calling-time -the-nations-drinking-as-a-major-health-issue/ (last accessed 18 March 2015).

Barbash, G.I. and Glied, S.A. (2010). New technology and health care costs – the case of robot-assisted surgery. *New England Journal of Medicine*, **363**(8), 701–704.

Barnett, K., Mercer, S.W., Norbury, M. *et al.* (2012). Research paper. Epidemiology of multi-morbidity and implications for health care, research and medical education: a cross-sectional study. *Lancet*, **380**(9836), 37–43.

Blustein, D. (2006). *The Psychology of Working: A New Perspective for Career Development, Counseling and Public Policy.* Taylor and Francis: London.

Burke, F.J., Main, J.R. and Freeman, R. (1997). The practice of dentistry: an assessment for premature retirement. *British Dental Journal*, **182**, 250–254.

Cho, J.Y., Lim, S.M. and Lim, J.Y. (2014). Targeted therapy in gastric cancer: personalizing cancer treatment based on patient genome. *World Journal of Gastroenterology*, **20**(8), 2042–2050.

Gale, E.N. (1998). Stress in dentistry. *New York State Dental Journal*, **64**, 30–34.

Gilmour, J., Stewardson, D.A., Shugars, D.A. and Burke, F.J.T. (2005). An assessment of career satisfaction among a group of general dental practitioners in Staffordshire. *British Dental Journal*, **198**, 701–704.

Gorter, R., Albrecht, G., Hoogstraten, J. and Eijkman, M. (1998). Work place characteristics, work stress and burnout among Dutch dentists. *European Journal of Oral Science*, **106**, 999–1005.

Health and Social Care Information Centre. (2011). Executive Summary: Adult Dental Health Survey 2009. Available from: http://www.dhsspsni.gov.uk/adhexecutive summary.pdf (last accessed 18 March 2015).

Humphris, G. (1999). Improved working conditions and professional support will benefit young dentists. *British Dental Journal*, **186**, 25.

Kay, E.J. and Lowe, J.C. (2008). A survey of stress levels, self-perceived health and health-related behaviors of UK dental practitioners in 2005. *British Dental Journal*, **204**, E19.

Kay, E. and Scarrott, D.M. (1997). A survey of dental professionals' health and well-being. *British Dental Journal*, **183**, 340–345.

King's Fund. (2012). Transforming the delivery of health and social care. *The case for fundamental change.* Available from: http://www.Kingsfund.org.uk/think (last accessed 18 March 2015).

Myers, H.L. and Myers, L.B. (2004). 'It's difficult being a dentist': stress and health in the general dental practitioner. *British Dental Journal*, **197**, 89–93.

Newbury-Birch, D., Lowry, R.J. and Kamali, F. (2002). The changing patterns of drinking, illicit drug use, stress, anxiety and depression in dental students in a UK dental school: a longitudinal study. *British Dental Journal*, **192**, 646–649.

OECD. (2013). Pensions at a glance 2013: OECD and G20 indicators. Available from: 10.1787/pension_glance-2013-en (last accessed 18 March 2015).

Office for National Statistics. (2012). Population estimates for the United Kingdom 27 March 2011. Available from: http://www.ons.gov.uk/ons/rel/census/2011-census/population-and-household-estimates-for-the-united-kingdom/stb-2011-census--population-estimates-for-the-united-kingdom.html#tab-Introduction (last accessed 18 March 2015).

Ramsden, R. (2013). *More people delaying retirement than last year.* Available from: http://www.saga.co.uk/newsroom/press-releases/2013/november/more-people-delaying-retirement-than-last-year.aspx (last accessed 18 March 2015).

Snell, T., Wittenberg, R., Fernandez, J.-L., *et al.* (2011). Projections of demand for social care and disability benefits for younger adults in England. Report of research conducted for the Commission on Funding of Care and Support. Economics of Social and Health Care Research Unit, discussion paper 2800/03. Available from: http://www.pssru.ac.uk/pdf/DP2880-3.pdf (last accessed 18 March 2015).

Stewart, F.M.J, Drummond, J.R, Carson, L. and Theaker, E.D. (2007). Senior dental students' career intensions, work-life balance and retirement plans. *British Dental Journal*, **203**, 257–263.

Super, D.E., Savickas, M.L. and Super, C.M. (1996). The life-span, life-space approach to careers. In: Brown, D. and Brooks, L. (eds). Career Choice and Development, 3rd edn. Jossey-Bass: San Francisco, CA, pp. 121–178.

Wang, Z., Klipfell, E., Bennett, B.J., *et al.* (2011). Gut flora metabolism of phosphatidylcholine promotes cardiovascular disease. *Nature*, **472**(7341), 57–63.

Wieder, M., Faigenblum, M., Eder, A. and Louca, C. (2013). An investigation of complete denture teaching in the UK: Part 1. A survey of undergraduate teaching. *British Dental Journal*, **215**, 177–181.

Willet, J. and Palmer, O.A. (2009). An investigation of the attitudes and fears of vocational dental practitioners in England and Wales in 2007. *Primary Dental Care*, **16**, 103–110.

Chapter 3 **Dental opportunities**

```
P  R  O  F  I  L  E                        M
            E  A        D  I  V  E  R  S  I  F  Y
      G     A           E                 X     E
      O  P  P  O  R  T  U  N  I  T  I  E  S     S
      A        N        T                 K
      L        E        A        N        I
      S     T  R  A  N  S  L  A  T  E     L
                        W        E        L
                                          S
```

> *Top Tip: Get involved*
>
>   Janine Brooks

Is the dental workforce today the workforce we will need in 10–20 years and beyond?

I doubt that the answer to this question is 'Yes'. I would also venture that it shouldn't be. Our patients are changing, society constantly changes, dentistry changes and so do we, the dental professionals. I suggest to you that the dental workforce needed in 10–20 years' time is not going to be the same one needed today. That is almost certainly true in respect to the skills required and the composition of the workforce. With that in mind, your career will need to be flexible enough to allow you to remain employed in dentistry (should you wish to be). One way to ensure this is to develop a career portfolio.

What about skill mix? Good thing or bad thing? I strongly feel it's a good thing: the patients benefit and we, the dental professionals, benefit. Across the globe, and certainly across Europe, the United Kingdom has the advantage of having one of the largest dental teams with regard to categories of staff. If we play to each others' strengths, we can provide more effective care to our patients and increase job satisfaction for each other.

How to Develop Your Career in Dentistry, First Edition. Janine Brooks.
© 2015 John Wiley & Sons, Ltd. Published 2015 by John Wiley & Sons, Ltd.

> **Top Tip:** *Don't be afraid to try new things*
>
> Debbie White

We are in a unique position in that we see patients from across age groups, many of whom do not regularly attend their doctors. People usually only go to see their doctor when something seems to be wrong. Dental professionals see patients who are well (or think they are), and that gives us the opportunity to be at the forefront of disease prevention and wellness. Dental professions can provide patients with smoking cessation classes, tests for diabetes and blood-pressure assessments. Why not? We regularly bemoan the fact that our skills are not properly recognised across general health care. We regularly try to make health colleagues and patients understand that good oral health impacts on good general health. We know that the mouth can show pointers to general health issues and systemic disease.

My predictions for the future are:
- Fewer dentists, who undertake the most challenging treatments.
- More DCPs, who undertake more routine dental treatments.
- More expanded-duties dental nurses, who use their skills and run dedicated patient sessions for:
  - oral hygiene instruction; and
  - diet advice.
- Dental practices offering additional patient services, such as:
  - smoking cessation; and
  - specialist tests: diabetic, cholesterol, blood pressure checks.

> **Career Highlight:** *Publishing my first book*
>
> Derek Richards

How can I develop a portfolio career?

The answer, of course, is 'In many ways'. In this section, I give you a few ideas on ways of building and developing your career into a portfolio.

Tips
- Learn your dental craft.
- Build your network and nurture it.
- Get more qualifications.
- Get involved and build your skills.
- Start to diversify.
- It's not just about dentistry – think widely.

- Learn to translate.
- It's never too late.
- Know yourself better.

Learn your dental craft

This is about spending time learning your profession, getting the basics well and truly cracked: honing your practical clinical skills, your communication skills, moving from a beginner to a mature, confident professional. This is the foundation for your future. It gives you credibility, experience and a solid base from which to diversify. Plan to spend 5–10 years really learning your craft; it will pay dividends later. It helps to move around a bit, although not so much that you never settle long enough to learn. Work in different sectors of dentistry, different practices – you'll learn what works and what doesn't, and your confidence will blossom.

Build your network and nurture it

I can't emphasise enough how vital networks are, and not just because they help with work opportunities. When I say your networks keep you sane, I mean it with all my heart. I learnt from my very early days in dentistry that networks are essential and important. My first dental boss, a District Dental Officer in Herefordshire, strongly encouraged me to attend dental meetings, both at our local Herefordshire Dental Society and the West Midlands BDA group meetings. He said I should get to know my dental colleagues, local and regional. These were the people I would work with and who would help me in my career. And how right he was. Not only did he encourage me to make the 100+ mile round trip up to Birmingham for meetings and to attend the local Herefordshire meetings, he often attended them himself. He made sure I knew who was who and why I should get to know them. Getting to know my local colleagues from general practice and the hospital service made my working life much easier. I knew who to make referrals to, who specialised in what, who to ask if I had a query about a patient or a clinical issue. I know my patients benefited from the good professional networks I built with my colleagues. Building my regional networks helped increase my political knowledge and skills. I quickly learnt that there was far more to dentistry than clinical care. Later, when I started my Masters in Community Dental Health course at Birmingham Dental School, my closest network took shape. I still regularly meet with four of my fellow students from those days; they have supported me through thick and thin. I can honestly say that without their unwavering personal and professional support, I wouldn't have achieved half of what I have.

Network, network, network, and if in doubt, network – more on that in Chapter 6.

Keep contact details for colleagues you meet and build your LinkedIn profile. It's important to make the most of the skills and experience you have. I don't mean overdoing it, but many dental professionals are poor at understanding or appreciating the nonclinical skills they have. Yes, most of us are clinicians, but we are all so much more.

Top Tip: *Accept tasks and jobs outside your comfort zone, or else you will stagnate rather than grow*

Janet Clarke

Get more qualifications

I'm sure you know this, but your basic dental qualification is just the beginning. Actually, for some, the beginning may well have started BD – Before Dentistry. I was a Medical Laboratory Technician working in haematology and cytogenetics before I saw the light and began my dental studies.

Gaining more qualifications opens the door to new opportunities. These obviously need to be paired with skill and experience to have maximum benefit, so that you can really build your portfolio and diversify your career.

What sort of qualifications are available? The answer is as diverse as the diversity of dentistry. Some will be obvious 'dental' qualifications, such as a Masters in Endodontics or an Advanced Certificate in Aesthetic Dentistry. Others will be nonclinical, such as health informatics or coaching, but their impact will mean you develop a more interesting profile. You will most likely have to pay for the longer courses, but it's investing in your future. These days, the format of courses and qualifications is wide, ranging from full-time courses to distance learning to blended online/tutored qualifications. There is something to suit most peoples' lifestyles and commitments. You can find out more about training and qualifications in Chapter 7.

Get involved and build your skills

You might think this is about networking, and it is, but it's more than that. It's about gaining experience, expertise and skills and developing yourself, particularly in nonclinical areas. If you think clinical skills are the only skills worth having in dentistry, think again. Some might suggest nonclinical skills are even more important. Getting involved in dental and non-dental work is an important aspect of preparing for and building a portfolio career. Getting involved means saying 'Yes'. 'Yes' to serving on a committee, 'Yes' to project managing a new development in your practice or organisation, 'Yes' to being a trainer. Often it may not be obvious how it will aid your career: career development is not always linear; in fact, it probably almost always isn't. If you know how to, you can gain from most of what you do.

These are the opportunities that you don't learn about at dental school, but that build your skills in communication, leadership, management and politics. For example, working on a committee can strengthen your negotiation capability.

> **Top Tip:** *Make the most of opportunities*
>
> Derek Richards

Start to diversify

When you begin to diversify, you'll probably want to start small – perhaps one day a week. It might feel like quite a challenge, being a bit out of your comfort zone. However, if you persevere, it will be worth it. Alternatively, you could become a committee member, perhaps on your local BDA branch or your Local Dental Committee (LDC). Both are good ways to build new skills and learn about what's happening in the wider dental world and in health care. Other opportunities you might want to think about are being a foundation trainer or a Deanery tutor, or giving presentations/lectures. Some useful preparation would be to take a short course on presentations skills or how to use PowerPoint. It's always a good idea to go and talk with your local dental dean or dental school about what might be available. Now would be a good time to think about adding some new qualifications to your repertoire, such as a Certificate in Medical Education.

Some opportunities you can take in addition to the day job, at evenings and weekends, which is great for dipping your toe into something new and finding out what you enjoy doing or what you want to do more of. Some jobs you will need to make room for. By that I mean, reducing your clinical commitment, perhaps from five days to four. A few people get the portfolio bug and slowly make more and more time for fresh opportunities.

It's not just about dentistry – think widely

Sometimes we dental professionals can be a bit focused on dentistry and miss out on the opportunities in wider health care, higher education and beyond. For those who work in salaried services or secondary care, these opportunities are often a bit more obvious and easier to take advantage of. What sort of thing do I mean? Opportunities like general management, project management, information governance, task groups. The advantages are that you widen the skills you have, you broaden your contacts and networks and you can reuse the skills you learn in dentistry (see next section). I worked for a time as an external verifier for City & Guilds and I learnt a lot about quality assurance, assessment tools, accreditation and benchmarking, all of which I've recycled within dentistry numerous times. I've worked as a facilitator/assessor for the Institute of Healthcare

Management, and that opened my eyes to reflective learning, reflective models and the underpinning theories. I realised that much of the reflection undertaken in dentistry is rather superficial, shallow and descriptive; in fact, not really reflection at all. Another advantage in taking a step outside dentistry is the people you meet and the ideas they expose you to. We dental professionals can be an isolated lot, so it can be a revelation to see how other professionals view the world and the great ideas they have. You have to learn to not get hung up on whether something has 'dental' written on it. As you build your portfolio, it can be the non-dental experiences that help you to stand out from the crowd and give you the edge when applying for jobs.

Career Highlight: *Steele Review*

Janet Clark

Learn to translate

I wrote in the previous section that some dental professionals need to see 'dental' attached to a topic, document or piece of work before they see the relevance of it. Over the years, I've come to realise this means you can miss out on useful information, ways of working and opportunities. You need to become adept at translating general into dental. When I go to non-dental conferences or lectures, I spend a lot of the time thinking, 'How can I use this?' 'How does this translate to dentistry?' 'How can I adapt this?' You know the answer: it's that most useful tools, techniques and models can be refreshed and applied to dentistry and dental professionals.

It's never too late

You can build your portfolio at any stage of your career, and the longer you have worked in dentistry, the easier you may find it. You will have more experience, you will have developed more skills and your confidence in your own abilities should be well developed. Of course, sometimes the reverse can feel true and you may need the support of a coach or mentor. In Chapter 2, I wrote about age bands and what people of different ages were looking for in their careers. As we travel through the age bands, our ability to expand our career increases, and we can achieve a varied portfolio of professional interests and roles. I have also written that I believe full retirement to be a concept that is undergoing radical change; therefore, older professionals may find this the perfect time to take a further qualification and become an adviser, expert witness, coach, mentor or inspector. It's never too late.

Know yourself better

In thinking about your career, whether you are at the beginning, at a crossroads or feel you have plateaued, you will find it useful to consider what you want from your life. You should think about what has brought you to where you are, what makes you what you are (e.g. your skills, strengths, weaknesses, interests, values and attitudes). This helps you understand the resources you have to help take your career forward. Now you must think about making the best of what you have and what you are. Each of us has a unique combination of skills, attitudes and experiences, and you need to use these to your best ability.

The first two steps will have helped you learn more about yourself and form the base for your personal development plan. The next step is the action plan: What are you going to do to achieve your goal?

When making decisions about your career, there are five steps that can help:

1. Think about your career goals.
2. Think about what routes you can take.
3. Decide what you need to get where you want to go.
4. Develop your skills.
5. Get prepared.

Thinking about your goals should take you some time. Coaching can help here: a coach will support you to explore and clarify what your goals are, to set your vision for your future. The route map and the tools you need are steps that a mentor can help you with. You can find more information about both coaching and mentoring in Chapter 4. Skill development will include qualifications, training and experience. I have covered aspects of each of these in Chapter 7.

> **Top Tip:** *Learning is lifelong and you will never stop learning*
> Shazad Malik

Dental careers – variety and opportunity

In Table 3.1, I list some of the main aspects or branches of dental careers alongside the more common subdivisions or roles. In this section, I provide a brief overview of some of these aspects, along with some personal accounts of specific roles from dental professionals working within them.

General practice (primary care)

Approximately 90–95% of dental care is provided in primary care settings, whether by nonsalaried general dental practitioners (GDPs), salaried GDPs, private practitioners or Community Dental Service (CDS) practitioners.

Most nonsalaried GDS dentists provide both NHS and private treatments; this is known as a 'mixed practice'. The proportion of NHS to private care provided by any one dentist varies from 1 to 99%. A small number of dentists provide either wholly NHS or wholly private practice. Where a dentist

Table 3.1 Major aspects of dentistry and their subdivisions

Aspect of dentistry	Subdivisions or roles
General practice (primary care)	Owner/principal
	Associate – performer/provider
	Corporate body
NHS	Foundation Trainer (FT)/Vocational Trainer (VT)
Private	Prison dentistry
	Appraiser
Salaried practice (primary care)	Special care
	Community dental
	Clinical director
Social enterprise	FT/VT trainer
	Prison dentists
	Appraiser
Secondary/specialty	Orthodontics
	Oral surgery
	Dental and maxillofacial radiology
Hospital	Dental public health
Community	Oral and maxillofacial pathology
General practice	Oral medicine
Social enterprise	Oral microbiology
	Restorative dentistry
	Endodontics
	Periodontology
	Paediatric dentistry
	Prosthodontics
	Special care
Armed Forces	Acting captain
	Captain
	Major
	Lieutenant colonel
	Colonel
Academia	Dental school
	Clinical academics
	Professor
	Clinical reader
	Clinical senior lecturer
	Clinical lecturer
Research	All dental schools have research departments
	Most academic dentists are involved in research as well as in teaching
Adviser/assessor	Medicolegal – indemnity (DPS, DDU. MDDUS)
	Dental practice – NHS England, NHS Scotland, NHS Wales, Health & Social Care Board NI
	Performance – National Clinical Assessment Service
	Regulatory – GDC, CQC
	Educational – Health Education England, GDC
	Charities – Bridge2Aid

Table 3.1 (*continued*)

Aspect of dentistry	Subdivisions or roles
Education/training	Postgraduate deanery (Health Education England)
	Tutor
	Lecturer
	External examiner
	Examiner
	FT trainer
	Dental Core Training trainer
Dental politics	British Dental Association (BDA)
	Local Dental Network (LDN)
	Committee member – specialist societies
	Department of Health
Regulation	GDC – fitness to practice, investigating committee
	Educational inspector
	CQC
	Expert witness
Management	Dental field – non-executive director, chairman
	Health field – chief executive
Development/support	Coach
	Mentor
	Appraiser
Dental journalism	Editor, contributor
Dental volunteer	Short – long-term overseas work
Dental historian	BDA
	Society of apothecaries
	Writer, researcher

provides NHS treatment, they are required, under their contract with the NHS, to offer treatment that is necessary to secure and maintain their patient's oral health. The amount of private work any dentist undertakes will depend upon the willingness and ability of their patients to meet the costs of their procedures.

To work in NHS dentistry, a dentist must be on a performer list (Health Board in Scotland, NHS England in England, NHS Wales in Wales; in Northern Ireland, a dentist must be entered on the Family Practitioner Services (FPS) dental list maintained by the Business Services Organisation). To be on a performer list, the dentist must have a Vocational Training (VT) number. To gain a VT number, the dentist must have successfully completed a Foundation (or Vocational) training year. Other groups of dental professionals do not need to be on a performer list.

Career Highlight: Being a Foundation dental trainer

Shazad Malik

Foundation Training/Vocational Training

Some dental practitioners are exempt from the requirement to complete dental FT/VT because:

- they are from a European Economic Area (EEA) Member State (other than the United Kingdom) and hold a recognised European Dental Diploma;
- they have had an NHS board or performer number within the last 5 years;
- they have practised in primary dental care in the CDS or the Armed Forces for 4 years full time (or equivalent part time), and for not less than 4 months during the past 4 years;
- they have completed a course of VT under the voluntary scheme; or
- their experience or training during the previous 5 years is equivalent to DFT.

A small number of newly qualified dentists do not enter FT/ VT and seek a position in private dentistry. Those who do so cannot obtain an NHS contract at any point in their subsequent career. The only way to do that is to have obtained a VT number.

There is a route, known as Foundation Training by Equivalence (FTE), whereby dentists without a VT number may attain equivalence to VT and thus obtain a VT number. This is a difficult path, as the dentist must secure a training practice and trainer (approved by their local deanery) that agrees to supervise them for 1 year, full time (or, occasionally, part time for 2 years). During that time, the FTE trainee attends offsite training as directed by the deanery and completes a portfolio of evidence. The portfolio, once submitted, will be assessed against criteria set by the deanery. If satisfactory, the postgraduate dental dean will award a VT number to the trainee and they may then apply to join a performers list and work within the NHS.

If a dentist ends his or her contract, perhaps to take a career break, and then wishes to rejoin the dental list, he or she needs to have a VT number before doing so.

Several postgraduate deaneries provide foundation training programmes for newly qualified dental therapists.

General dental practitioner

A clinical dentist works exclusively with patients. A day is likely to be 7–8 hours, if full time, with morning and afternoon sessions of 3–4 hours. Generally, a lunch break is taken. However, the needs and interests of the patients are paramount, so if a patient arrives late, there is an emergency or a treatment takes longer than expected, sessions can run over. Many dentists still work in single-chair practices as single practitioners, but most now work with colleagues. Corporate bodies have expanded since legal restrictions were removed, and they employed approximately 11% of the workforce across the United Kingdom in 2014. Dentists work with a dental nurse, who assists and supports the treatment provided.

Clinical dentists in general practice are operating a business. Their patients are their client base and, as with any service industry business, it is vital that they ensure customer satisfaction. Patients can, and do, change practice if they are dissatisfied with the quality of the service provided to them. Accordingly, it is vital that any dentist who works for a practice is not only competent but reliable. Patients will not, for obvious reasons, easily tolerate a situation where their dentist fails to turn up to treat them or curtails treatment because of illness.

Most dentists in practice see an average of 15–20 patients in a half-day session, with little time between each. Accordingly, in a full day, many dentists will see up to 40 patients. They will often engage in complex procedures that require considerable concentration. In addition to the clinical aspects, a dentist in general practice must be able to run their business, employ staff, use information technology, understand the legal underpinnings of dentistry and health care, understand finance and market their services appropriately.

General dental practice differs across the United Kingdom. The system in Scotland and Northern Ireland is not the same as that in England and Wales. In Scotland and Northern Ireland, dentists working in general practice can be nonsalaried (independent contractors) or salaried. NHS boards may employ salaried dentists to provide an alternative service to that of independent GDPs where there is a local shortage of dentists to provide NHS treatment. In addition, the CDS provides NHS care for patients with medical problems, patients with special needs and other disadvantaged groups who cannot use general dental services. Dentists who work in nonsalaried practice will be either principals or associates. A principal is a dental practitioner who is also an owner, director or partner of a dental practice and who has an arrangement with an NHS board to provide general dental services. An associate is a dental practitioner who is self-employed and enters into an arrangement with a principal dentist that is neither partnership nor employment; they also will have an arrangement with an NHS board to provide general dental services.

Career Highlight: Setting up my own dental practice

Shazad Malik

Box 3.1 General dental practitioner: Dr Malcolm Brady (private and NHS)

What does the job entail? I am a practice owner and work as a private dentist in that practice. I have worked in this practice for more than 20 years. This has allowed me to see the success and failure of the dental care I have carried out over the years. The experiences of my early years in NHS dentistry were occasionally demotivating. By that I mean providing treatment for patients who see no value in trying to retain their teeth, and watching restorative treatments fail in a short time due to lack of care on their part. There is no satisfaction in monitoring neglect. This was one of the reasons I wanted to practice privately. I wanted my patients to want their treatment, not just to need it. I realise this might sound dismissive of a large proportion of society, but it's not really. I do not treat millionaires or celebrities, just normal people who value their health sufficiently to want to pay for reliable care. I see patients with a broad spectrum of needs. I treat the majority myself and refer some to colleagues for specialist opinions or for certain types of treatment. My patients are mostly adults that require general restorative care. I have a strong emphasis on prevention, and promote hygiene and individual cleaning skills to patients who are well motivated to maintain and retain their teeth. I have a three-surgery practice and employ an associate and several part-time hygienists.

　Great bits? I like being a dentist. I like meeting my patients, diagnosing their problems and caring for them in a professional yet friendly way. My favourite type of treatment is endodontics. Management of the dental pulp is such a crucial aspect of most treatments. If you get this aspect of treatment wrong you will have many unhappy patients. I discovered early in my career that predictable management of vital teeth and reliable endodontic outcomes make happy patients who become regular long-term clients. If you want to charge significant fees for your expertise then the treatment you provide must be successful.

　Not so great bits? Managing a modern dental practice is a job in itself. Managing staff, employing them, motivating them and forming a strong team is difficult. Overseeing the culture of the practice and keeping everyone on track can be time consuming and draining. But it can also be very rewarding. You need a wide variety of personal skills to manage people in the workplace. You will come across many difficult circumstances when staff look to you for help, advice and leadership. There will inevitably be conflicts, which you may need to arbitrate. This is an area that we don't get much training in. However, when you get it right, and forge a successful team, you gain enormous satisfaction. Especially when that team begins to perpetuate the culture you have prescribed.

Do you have any special interests? I like restorative dentistry. It was very clear to me from early in my career that unless you can provide reliable endodontics you will not progress. So often this is the bedrock of a restorative case. I bought a dental microscope 15 years ago and use it for all my work, even examinations. The vision it gives you is amazing. I recommend you try it. I joined the British societies of specialties I was interested in, for example, the British Endodontic Society. This is a group of like-minded dentists who want to provide the best. It is a society full of endodontic specialists but it also has hundreds of GDPs who want to improve their skills. Joining such societies and attending their meetings is an excellent way to up-skill yourself without going down the postgraduate degree route. I also do a fair amount of orthodontics. The way the current NHS dental contract is written prevents GDPs from doing any orthodontics and this is a great shame. Restorative care can be greatly enhanced by the addition of orthodontic skills. Cases can be treated far more conservatively and with much less intervention. I would advise anyone to gain experience in this field if they can.

Did you take further qualifications to practice your special interest? If so, what are they? I joined the Central London Study Group soon after qualifying and I would urge anyone to find something similar and sign up. Preparation for the Faculty of General Dental Practice (FGDP) membership exams is a very useful starting point for any career. There are lots of short courses available these days, which are excellent if you want to stay in general practice and develop your operative skills.

Top tips Learn to be confident. Communicate clearly with patients and write your notes very thoroughly.

Top Tip: Be willing to help others

Sophie Noske

Box 3.2 Dental corporate – area clinical manager/clinical support manager: Dr Manish Chitnis

What qualifications did you need for this job? *Mandatory:* GDC registered dentist with an NHS performer number. Working in NHS for more than 4 years with extensive experience in the working regulations of the NHS. *Desirable:* Certificate or diploma in dental practice management (e.g. Bristol University).

What does the job entail? Facilitation between the operations team and the clinical team. Clinical audit, recruitment interviews, Continuing Professional Development (CPD) facilitation, Personal Development Plan (PDP) facilitation and guidance, monthly peer reviews and newsletter information, helping dentists in difficulty, induction and training for dentists new to the NHS, direct observation of clinical work, working on clinical and related business growth of clinicians, education support, exit of dentists for nonperformance and gross misconduct, managing and resolving patient clinical complaints and providing support to the operation team in drafting responses.

Great bits? The opportunity to learn, share and see the positive growth of the clinical group. Communication with different peers and the complete experience of running a dental business. It has matured me as a clinician and my knowledge of business management has been a steep learning curve.

Not so great bits? The travel involved in this job – sometimes 200 miles to meet someone for a 30-minute meeting! Technology has helped and remote access (Skype etc.) is helping manage distances now.

Top tips You need passion to help people and to have a genuine interest in the positive growth of your peers. You need a balance of understanding for the conflict between clinicians and the operational team to make a decision in favour of everybody's best interest. Dental corporates have their own business strategies and you need to work with the best interests in the following order:

1. the patient;
2. the performing team; and
3. the business.

If you don't get this sequence right you will get frustrated with your decision-making as a clinical lead in a corporate!

Box 3.3 Foundation dentist trainer: Dr Shazad Malik

What qualifications did you need for this job? BDS.

What does the job entail? Being a supervisor, mentor, teacher, friend and boss to a newly graduated dentist.

Great bits? The role is very challenging, with you constantly juggling your various hats from being a supervisor to teacher throughout the year. By providing a rich learning environment you get to see the new graduate grow into an advanced safe beginner.

Not so great bits? The stress of having to deal with fall out with patients when things go wrong.

Top tips Have lots of patience and enjoy your time, it will go very quickly. Before you know it, the foundation dentist will be ready to fly the nest.

Salaried practice

Salaried primary dental care dental professionals can work in CDSs or in a social enterprise. The names given to the grades of job role within salaried primary dental care differ across the United Kingdom: Table 3.2 lists different roles and gives their equivalent across the country; for example, a Foundation dentist working in England, Wales or Northern Ireland is in the same job grade as a Vocational dentist working in Scotland; a Band C Clinical dentist undertakes the same job grade as an associate specialist.

> **Top Tip:** *Everybody is equal, no one is superior – they are just at a different stage of their career*
>
> Bal Chana

Table 3.2 Comparison of job grade categories

Job grade	Combined categories
Foundation dentist DF1	Foundation dentist DF1/DF2
Foundation dentist DF2	Vocational dentist (Scotland)
Band A	Band A/dental officer/salaried GDP
Dental officer	
Salaried GDP	
Band B	Band B/senior dental officer/senior
Senior dental officer	salaried GDP
Senior salaried GDP	
Band C Clinical	Band C Clinical/associate specialist
Associate specialist	
Band C Managerial	Band C Managerial/Clinical
Clinical director	Director/assistant clinical
Assistant clinical director	Director/CADO
Clinical administrative dental officer	
Consultant	Consultant
Other	

Box 3.4 Specialist – special care dentistry: Dr Heather Pope

What qualifications did you need for this job? BDS to start then post-graduate experience in maxillofacial/oral surgery to broaden and deepen skills gained during the undergraduate period. Clinical experience in routine and paediatric dentistry gained via a CDS post, gradually incorporating more complex special needs patient care.

Increasing clinical experience and knowledge of service management/development gained via a postgraduate masters degree (MCDH). At the same time, a DDPHRCS, securing future access to the Royal College structures. Just as important as these formal qualifications is the learned ability to appear calm no matter what happens and to remain patient throughout difficult appointments.

What does the job entail? Clinical assessment and treatment of all types and ages of special needs patients. This includes people with physical, cognitive, sensory, emotional and social impairments. People with complex medical histories and those who have undergone extensive surgery following trauma or head/neck cancer. In addition: development of services to meet the needs of these varied patients; education and training of care staff to ensure ongoing oral health for their clients; training and development of dental staff to enable them to contribute to treatment services; liaison with a wide network of health and social care professionals to ensure that all dental treatment is safe and appropriate to the individual patient.

Great bits? Patient contact and the daily histories, stories and conversations that we have with them and their carers. Seeing their oral health improvement, often from a very poor starting point.

Not so great bits? The frustrations of working within large NHS organisations, where progress and development can seem slow.

Top tips Only consider this type of career if you genuinely enjoy interaction with all groups of people in difficult circumstances! Gain experience in general dentistry and oral surgery before starting to work with these challenging patients. You often have only a very brief timeframe in which to achieve a lasting, definitive result.

Secondary care/specialty dentistry

All secondary care dental specialties are commissioned by NHS England. The actual work can be carried out in hospital settings or primary care (i.e. general practice, community services or social enterprises). Many services are consultant-led. Dental hospitals also provide secondary care and are an important part of training for the specialties.

Specialist lists

The GDC recognises 13 dental specialties. Each requires successful completion of a training pathway. A relatively small number of dental professionals enter specialty training: less than 10% of dentists on the dental register are specialists in the recognised categories. Table 3.3 lists the specialties and the numbers of dentists registered with the GDC for each at the end of 2013.

At 31 December 2013, there were a total of 4339 dentists registered as specialists. About a quarter of these were orthodontists. Clearly, if your heart is set upon being an oral microbiologist, you will have to accept there are not many jobs available.

A number of the specialties require direct patient contact (i.e. intervention care and treatment), while others are less directly patient contact-focused. Of the 13 specialties, the following 5 fall into that category:

- dental and maxillofacial radiology;
- dental public health;
- oral and maxillofacial pathology (essentially laboratory work);
- oral medicine; and
- oral microbiology.

Regardless of the degree of direct patient contact, all require considerable further training on consultant career pathways. The training pathways vary in length from 5–10 years from leaving dental school to successful completion of a specialty training programme and the award of a Certificate of Completion of Specialist Training (CCST). Part of that training pathway

Table 3.3 Number of dentists registered by specialty, 31 December 2013

Dentist specialty	Count
Dental and maxillofacial radiology	25
Dental public health	119
Endodontics	260
Oral and maxillofacial pathology	32
Oral medicine	76
Oral microbiology	7
Oral surgery	765
Orthodontics	1383
Paediatric dentistry	247
Periodontics	343
Prosthodontics	440
Restorative dentistry	317
Special care dentistry	325
TOTAL FOR ALL SPECIALTIES	**4339**

Source: General Dental Council.

will be to work directly with patients. After a CCST has been attained, it is anticipated that holders will need to gain post-CCST experience and further competences before applying for a consultant post. Therefore, a realistic timeframe is 10–15 years from leaving dental school to becoming a consultant, if you begin your training as soon as you are able. Obviously, some people work in dentistry for some years before deciding to enter specialist training. Health Education England (HEE) was established as a Special Health Authority in June 2012. Dentistry is one of seven HEE advisory bodies. HEE is accountable for English issues only; NHS Education Scotland (NES) in Scotland and postgraduate deaneries in Northern Ireland and Wales have similar lead roles. Postgraduate deans are responsible for specialty training programmes. The deaneries work with the Royal Colleges and faculties to manage quality postgraduate training. The specialties each have their own societies, which are a good source of information if you are thinking of expanding your career in this direction.

The following list provides a brief outline of what each speciality entails; the descriptions are informed by the GDC definitions of dental specialties:

1. **Dental public health:** This is a nonclinical specialty involving the science and art of preventing oral diseases by promoting oral health to the population rather than the individual. It involves the assessment of dental health needs and ensuring dental services meet those needs.

2. **Oral medicine:** Oral medicine is concerned with the oral health care of patients who have chronic recurrent and medically related disorders of the mouth. It covers their diagnosis and nonsurgical management. It requires direct patient contact in specialist clinics.

3. **Oral microbiology:** Oral microbiologists diagnose and assess facial infection – typically bacterial and fungal disease. It is a clinical specialty undertaken by laboratory-based personnel, who provide reports and advice based on interpretation of microbiological samples. Direct contact with patients is minimal.

4. **Oral and maxillofacial pathology:** Oral and maxillofacial pathologists diagnose and make assessments from tissue changes characteristic of disease of the oral cavity, jaws and salivary glands. This is a clinical specialty undertaken by laboratory-based personnel. Direct contact with patients is minimal.

5. **Dental and maxillofacial radiology:** Dental and maxillofacial radiology involves all aspects of medical imaging, providing information about the anatomy, function and disease states of the teeth and jaws. It requires direct patient contact.

6. **Endodontics:** Specialists in endodontics study and treat disease and injury of the roots of teeth, dental pulp and surrounding tissues.

They undertake root canal therapy and other endodontic surgery, such as apicectomy.

7. **Oral surgery:** Specialists in oral surgery undertake complex surgical procedures unsuitable for general practice. These include complex extractions, irregularities and pathology of the jaw and mouth and minor trauma or major surgery with the use of general anaesthesia. Oral surgery does not require a medical degree. The specialty was previously called 'surgical dentistry'.

8. **Restorative dentistry:** This deals with the study, diagnosis and restoration to normal function of diseased, injured or abnormal teeth. Restorative dentistry encompasses the specialties of endodontics, periodontics and prosthodontics. It integrates care for patients with complex treatment needs resulting from developmental or acquired orofacial and dental diseases and conditions, as well as patients who have medical problems or learning difficulties that have implications for their care.

9. **Orthodontics:** This is the development, prevention and correction of irregularities of the teeth, bite and jaws.

10. **Paediatric dentistry:** Specialists in paediatric dentistry provide care and treatment for child patients – generally child patients who present with a challenge, including developmental abnormalities such as cleft lip and palate; illness, such as leukaemia; and special needs, such as Down syndrome. Dentists who get on well with children and enjoy working with them might find this specialty is for them.

11. **Special care dentistry:** This is concerned with the improvement of the oral health of individuals (children, adults and older adults) and groups in society who have a physical, sensory, intellectual, mental, medical, emotional or social impairment or disability, or, more often, a combination of these factors.

12. **Periodontics:** This involves the diagnosis, treatment and prevention of diseases and disorders (infections and inflammatory) of the gums and other structures around the teeth.

13. **Prosthodontics:** This involves the replacement of missing teeth and the associated soft and hard tissues by prostheses (crowns, bridges, dentures), which may be fixed or removable, or may be supported and retained by implants.

In any of the 13 dental specialties, including those with no direct patient contact, it is possible for a dental surgeon to pursue either a clinical or an academic role, and many combine both aspects in their career. Each specialty requires the individual to undertake additional training following their initial university course and qualification as a dentist. They all require applicants to have successfully completed a minimum of 2 years' postqualification training, including VT/FT prior to application to the specialist training programme. The specialist career pathways range from 3 to 5 years in length.

If a dentist wishes to become a specialist in the United Kingdom, they must complete a training programme approved by the GDC. The training programme is designed to lead to the award of a CCST. A dentist must hold full GDC registration to be awarded a CCST. Each CCST has specific entry, training and assessment criteria. The specialty curricula for each of the 13 specialities have been approved by the GDC and can be found at http://www.gdc-uk.org/Dentalprofessionals/Specialistlist/Pages/default.aspx (last accessed 18 March 2015). Once on a specialist GDC list, you may be able to take up a consultant post in the NHS. A few specialties require a further period of post-CCST training. The Royal Surgical Colleges award the specific qualification, while the postgraduate dental deans receive applications for approved training programmes and monitor dentists while they are completing their training.

The curricula for training in each specialty take their guidance from a number of documents. The Dental Gold Guide (COPDED, 2013) is a must read. It is produced by the UK Committee of Postgraduate Dental Deans and Directors (COPDEND) and is approved by the four UK Departments of Health. I recommend that, in addition, you read the requirements for the particular training programme you are interested in. The following are helpful references:

- The Postgraduate Medical Education and Training Board's (PMETB) Standards for Curricula.
- The PMETB's Principles for an Assessment System for Postgraduate Medical Training Principles for an Assessment System for Postgraduate Medical Training.
- The Faculty of Public Health of the Royal Colleges of Physicians of the United Kingdom Public Health Training Curriculum 2007.
- Medical leadership competency framework, jointly developed by the Academy of Medical Royal Colleges and NHS Institute for Innovation and Improvement.
- Skills for Health Career framework.

> **Top Tip:** *Keep learning*
>
> Janine Brooks

Less-than-full-time training

This used to be known as 'flexible training'. All of the dental specialty training programmes allow less-than-full-time training, which normally involves between five and eight sessions per week. The aim is to provide opportunities for dentists in the NHS who are unable to work full time. Dentists can apply for less-than-full-time training if they can provide evidence that 'training on a full-time basis would not be practicable for well-founded individual reasons' (COPDEND, 2013).

Many dental professionals will wish to develop their skills in a specialty area but prefer not to undertake full specialist training. They will want to expand their knowledge and experience. For those individuals, there are a range of training options with qualifications offered by the dental schools, although not every dental school offers postgraduate qualifications in all 13 specialty areas. Training programmes are also offered by private training organisations. Chapter 7 gives more details about the availability of training and qualifications.

Box 3.5 Trainee in dental public health: Dr Reena Patel

What qualifications did you need for this job? *Essential:* BDS or equivalent; full registration with GDC as a dentist; 2 years' foundation training (general professional training) or equivalent. *Desirable:* FDS/MFDS/ MJDF or equivalent; MPH/MSc DPH.

What does the job entail? The training post will allow the trainee to develop an appropriate level of knowledge and skill in the following curriculum areas:

- Oral health surveillance.
- Assessing the evidence on oral health and dental interventions, programmes and services.
- Policy and strategy development and implementation.
- Strategic leadership and collaborative working for health.
- Oral health improvement.
- Health and public protection.
- Developing and monitoring quality dental services.
- Dental public health intelligence.
- Academic dental public health.
- Appropriate decision-making and judgement.
- Appropriate attitudes, ethical understanding and legal responsibilities.
- Role within the health services.
- Personal development.

Great bits? The constant transition! DPH is a very political specialty, meaning that every change of government will no doubt bring a change in the structure of health and social care systems, and changes to the role of a dental public health consultant.

Not so great bits? Lack of job security. This is a real issue given that there are very limited job opportunities following a lengthy training programme, during which you become deskilled as a clinician.

Top tips Be flexible and open-minded … every day is a very different day.

Box 3.6 Hospital practitioner, orthodontics: Mr Peter Thornley

What qualifications did you need for this job? BDS and attendance at clinical assistant training courses.

What does the job entail? Carrying out orthodontic treatment under the direction of a consultant at the local hospital. Taking records, models and photographs before treatment starts, fitting fixed appliances for straightforward cases (e.g. moderate class 2 div 1 with moderate crowding).

Great bits? Learning orthodontic skills and diagnosis with a consultant present who could help if I ran into difficulties. I learnt enough to be able to carry out 80% of treatment required for my own patients in practice, learnt what I should avoid treating and was in a very safe environment. I now feel confident to take referrals for fixed orthodontic treatment.

Not so great bits? With time, more training became available for specialist orthodontists and there are now very few places for GDPs with special interest in a hospital setting. I still carry out a lot of orthodontics in practice and achieve good Peer Assessment Rating (PAR) scores, but have now stopped the hospital post.

Top tips Get involved in a local managed clinical network and get to know your local consultant. The funding arrangements in hospitals are much more difficult these days, and training pathways for dentists with special interest are no longer present, I think because in the early stages it takes more of the consultant's time. Also, relatively simple cases are no longer accepted for treatment in hospital. However, if you can build a good relationship with a consultant and maybe consider doing some voluntary sessions, there might still be a few opportunities.

Armed forces

The armed forces offer a career in primary dental care with the opportunity to take specialist qualifications, such as a masters degree. You can enter the forces while a dental student: undergraduate cadetships are available which allow you to pass officer selection and earn money while a student. The army pays your tuition fees and an annual salary during your last 3 years of study. You must be a British, Commonwealth or Irish citizen, studying in a UK university and in the last 3 years of your course. During this time, you will have the rank of second lieutenant. Once qualified, you will undertake officer commissioning at the Royal Military Academy, Sandhurst, where you will have the rank of acting captain. After that, you complete your foundation training with an army practice and trainer; once you have completed this, you will have the rank of captain. While in the army you can also learn fieldcraft, tactics and weapons handling. In addition, leadership and management training is available.

The army consists of regulars – full-time soldiers – and reservists – part-time soldiers. Both can work in the United Kingdom or overseas.

Up-to-date information can be found at www.army.mod.uk.

Academia

Clinical academic

Clinical academia includes research, teaching and clinical sessions, where appropriate. Dental academics are also involved in management, student assessment and examinations and committee work within their establishment. Dental academics usually work in a university post in a dental teaching establishment. Not all academic staff are clinically qualified, and some undertake research and teaching. Academic staff from all of the dental specialties are involved in education and teaching. The teaching aspect can include undergraduate, postgraduate and all categories of dental registrants. Not all academics are involved in every aspect – it will depend on the particular post. Honorary positions are a good way to test the water. You won't get paid but you will get valuable experience, personal satisfaction and development, and they can open the door to other opportunities.

Clinical work is usually an important part of the role of a clinical academic and many will have trained to become specialists and then consultants, providing consultant care for patients. Alongside this, supervision and training for staff in training grades will often be undertaken. Involvement in audit, peer review, appraisal and other clinical governance activities will also be expected.

Academic staff can become involved in course development and design and student recruitment. They may also have an opportunity to undertake management roles in their establishment. Tutoring and examining for the Royal Colleges can be undertaken, or they can get involved in dental politics and work with the Department of Health.

How do I get in?

- Foundation training.
- Broad experience in general practice, salaried service, hospital service.
- Master Faculty Dental Surgery.

- Higher degree, for example a PhD.
- Teaching qualification.
- Specialist training.

Box 3.7 Visiting professor: Professor Ken Eaton

What qualifications did you need for this role? Many publications in international peer-reviewed journals. An internationally recognised academic track record. Knowledge and skills in the area in which I was appointed

What does the role entail? Working in specific areas with the faculty in the university concerned. The time commitment varies over the years and, in my case, differs from university to university. Essentially, the university wants to use your expertise, but not full time. It's good to have recognition of your status as a professor but without the commitment of tenure.

Great bits The flexibility that the appointment offers. Currently I have three visiting or honorary chairs and, subject to successful grant applications, two more are in the pipeline. The opportunity to travel.

Not so great bits? No particular aspects.

Top tips Publish widely in international peer-reviewed journals. Attend many international education and research meetings and build up a wide network.

Top Tip: Present solutions, not problems

Reena Patel

Research

Research is an important aspect of all academic posts. This might be as a sole researcher or with other academics. Most of those who undertake research will first have obtained a higher degree, such as a PhD, a DDS or a DMed Eth; there are a number available. After that, researchers work on a variety of research topics. Projects generally need external funding and most dental academics need to regularly prepare grant applications. Following from the research, papers will be written for publication and presentations will be made at conferences.

Box 3.8 Honorary research fellow: Mr Peter Thornley

What qualifications did you need for this job? BDS and an interest in research. Some kind of postgraduate qualification could help. I joined a local research network at the university. A voluntary post, but together our group won the BDA Shirley Glastone-Hughes prize twice, which funded two practice-based research projects.

What does the job entail? Taking part in research projects. This can vary from just collecting data to helping design protocols. Carrying out an MSc usually involves a research dissertation, which can develop useful skills for those interested in research, such as critical appraisal. The MFGDP and MJDF examinations also used to include elements of critical appraisal.

Great bits? Interesting to take part in research and especially influence research in general practice. Getting some papers published with your name on them. Having some research on your CV can be a big benefit when applying for other jobs, such as a dental advisor or foundation trainer.

Not so great bits? Can be time-consuming and quite a commitment to carefully collect data when you are a busy GDP.

Top tips Meet with colleagues from your local dental hospital, try and build contacts with people interested in research. The dental faculties usually hold a research day once per year, where you can build networks and meet others who might be interested in research, and also get some ideas on how to do it.

Adviser

There are many different types of adviser undertaking different roles, including working with a Local Area Team or a number of key dental and health organisations. Advisers are employed by the GDC, NCAS, CQC, the Health Ombudsman and some deaneries. The indemnity organisations also employ advisers to support members. They all use their professional expertise, built up over the years, to aid the organisation in its role in dentistry.

Box 3.9 Professional panellist, GDC Dental Complaints Service (DCS): Mr Steve Brookes

What qualifications did you need for this job? None beyond registration as a dental professional, but it would be useful if you were still in general practice and up to date.

What does the job entail? Receive details in connection with an unresolved complaint relating to private care, read through ensuring that all the documents required are present. Make personal notes as required. Agree a convenient time for the panel to meet; this is usually at a hotel, often quite local. Attend meetings and assist the lay members, dentist and complainant to agree a resolution to the complaint (if possible). Write up notes and the agreed resolution (if any) and the recommendations of the panel to the dentist and complainant.

Great bits? As this work is voluntary, you really feel that you are giving something back. It's nice to be able to help the patient resolve a complaint without recourse to legal measures. It's very satisfying when the dentist and complainant are reasonable and the complaint is resolved to the satisfaction of all.

Not so great bits? Hard to fit in with minimum disruption to running a practice. Seeing patients that have, in your opinion, a justifiable complaint but failing to achieve a resolution: it reflects badly on the profession.

Top tips Be prepared to work for free. Be reasonable and fair in your opinion of the dentist's work: it's easy to get on your high horse and pretend that all dental care is gold standard all of the time; we all have days when we get it wrong.

Box 3.10 BDA Good Practice Assessor: Dr Shazad Malik

What qualifications did you need for this job? No formal qualifications but must be either a practice manager or a dentist that has an excellent understanding of the BDA Good Practice Scheme.

What does the job entail? Doing onsite assessments at dental practices that want to become members of the BDA Good Practice Scheme. A consultancy role, in a nut shell.

Great bits? The privilege to go and do onsite assessments at dental practices, which allows me to pick up good practice and bring this back into my own practice. Also, meeting colleagues from different parts of London.

Not so great bits? Stubborn or difficult people.

Top tips Have a clear understanding of the principles, purpose and processes of assessment and an eye for detail.

Education/training

This covers a wide range of opportunities. All dental registrants can become involved in teaching, either for their particular aspect of dentistry, across the profession or even more broadly. Dental professionals who teach may work as clinical academics in dental schools, hold part-time posts or work in other areas of dentistry; for example, combining general practice or salaried practice with a dental school post. Those who work in primary dental care, either in general or salaried practice, can be Foundation Trainers and guide new dentists in their first year in practice. Dental professionals also teach in non-dental-school universities, higher education establishments and colleges. The subjects they teach will range from clinical to nonclinical; for example, law and ethics, communication skills and leadership. Some dental professionals have established their own training companies and offer education in the form of seminars, presentations and online resources.

Top Tip: Get involved in local dental affairs

Debbie White

Box 3.11 Teacher, clinical dental technicians: Miss Jackie Arnold

What qualifications did you need for this job? A further adult education teaching certificate. Assessing and Internal Verification qualifications. A dental nursing qualification.

What does the job entail? Teaching clinical dental technicians about cross-infection, health and safety, equality and diversity and working as a team. I also teach the role of the GDC and how it applies to DCPs.

Great bits? Nice to mix with different members of the dental team and talk about job experiences and the different ways things can be taught.

Not so great? Some dental technicians think they are better than me and don't need me to teach them.

Top tips Follow what you want to do and do it.

Top Tip: Allow yourself time to get used to new things

Debbie White

Box 3.12 DCP tutor: Miss Bal Chana

What qualifications did you need for this job? Qualified dental hygienist and therapist. Teaching qualification, such as a Certificate in Medical Education.

What does the job entail? Implementation and delivery of education and training programmes for dental hygiene and therapy students and undergraduate dental (BDS) students.

Great bits? I enjoy the clinical aspect of this role, sharing my experiences with the students. Providing support and guidance, aiding their development.

Not so great bits? Not a 9–5 job.

Top tips Mentor a tutor and teach on a voluntary basis.

Top Tip: Be nice to people and smile; this applies to everyone you meet and work with

Janet Clarke

Box 3.13 Honorary lecturer: Mrs Jane Davies-Slowik

What qualifications did you need for this job? Masters in Community Dental Health (MCDH).

What does the job entail? Providing education to undergraduates at Birmingham Dental School on aspects of the dental public health part of the curriculum.

Great bits? Contact with the undergraduates and the Dental Public Health Department. Can choose which sessions to do.

Not so great bits? Lack of remuneration sometimes, but the benefits outweigh the disadvantages.

Top tips Make sure you have enough time to devote to this. Think about the professional and personal benefits – it's good for keeping up to date and also for your curriculum vitae.

Career Highlight: Being an examiner for orthodontic therapy at the Royal College of Surgeons

Sophie Noske

Box 3.14 Examiner MJDF: Mr Peter Thornley

What qualifications did you need for this job? A postgraduate qualification – at least the equivalent of the level for which you are examining, but a higher-level qualification is better.

What does the job entail? Attending examiner training, then writing questions, taking part in examination diets, supervising Objective Structured Clinical Examinations (OSCEs) and Structured Clinical Reasoning Examinations (SCRs).

Great bits? Great place to network and an interesting change to general practice. Can help to keep you up to date as you need to keep up with the current literature if you are writing exam questions. Can help further your career in other fields, such as dental advisor, foundation training.

Not so great bits? Can be time-consuming and requires commitment. Not paid, but usually travel expenses and a meal with other examiners are provided.

Top tips Maybe start by being involved as a mentor for a local study group (assuming you have passed the examination yourself). Apply to the college, be enthusiastic and get stuck in writing questions – your career will then progress. You could end up becoming the chief examiner.

Box 3.15 External examiner: Miss Bal Chana

What qualifications did you need for this job? As an examiner you are required to hold an appropriate academic post, usually at a senior level within a university or other teaching establishment. You must also have expertise in the required field.

What does the job entail? Providing assurance that the assessment system is fair and operated equitably, and ensuring comparability of the standards with other institutions. These appointments are generally for a 3–4 year period.

Great bits? Ensuring the required standard is met by future graduates. Seeing how other institutes deliver their training programmes.

Not so great bits? Time.

Top tips Have a mentor. Start as an internal examiner.

Box 3.16 Examiner – Diploma Special Care Dentistry: Mrs Jane Davies-Slowik

What qualifications did you need for this job? *Essential:* BDS; registration with the GDC. *Desirable:* Postgraduate qualification appropriate to the post, i.e. special care dentistry; Fellow or Member of FDS RCS England or appropriate basic science qualification.

What does the job entail? Mark module assignments; design module questions; develop module resources; examine the written and oral section of the examination for 2 days per year; attend an initial training event before examining for the first time; attend a refresher training event each year (1 day); attend two examiner panel meetings per year, usually 3 hours' duration, held at the Royal College of Surgeons (RCS); submit new assessment material for the multiple-short-answer paper and/or the oral elements to the exam.

What do you like most? The opportunity to use my clinical skills as a special care dentist in a different way. The chance to see the examinations from the other side!

What do you like least? Nothing as yet.

Top tips Give it a go! Take your chances.

Top Tip: Share what you've learned along the way – it's fun to watch students grow

Emma Worrell

Dental politics

Learning how the politics of dentistry works can be fascinating. There are many opportunities to get involved in local and/or national politics. You can pick up considerable experience by putting yourself forward for society committees, as well as the British Dental Association, an LDC or a Local Dental Professional Network (LDPN). If you disagree with the way dentistry works, get into the system and help to improve it – don't moan from the sidelines. Getting involved in dental politics can give you a wider, more strategic view of dentistry and a different perspective on your own practice.

Box 3.17 Local Dental Committee (LDC): Mrs Claudia Peace

What qualifications did you need for this role? Qualified, practicing dentist and included on the Performer's List for NHS England Local Area Team (LAT).

What does the job entail? Liaising with NHS England LAT on behalf of all NHS dentists in our local area, bimonthly evening committee meetings to discuss local dental issues with the local dental public health consultant, dental practice advisor, community dentists, local academics, consultants, deanery representatives and the chair of the LDPN. Other work includes helping develop clinical pathways and managed clinical networks, providing CPD events for constituents and holding quarterly meetings of the LDC Executive with the LAT Dental Commissioner. As treasurer, I also have responsibility for the LDC accounts and work closely with the LDC secretary, including representation at Area Team Performance Screening Groups, attendance at the annual national LDC conferences biannually and sitting on various subcommittees.

Great bits How much I have learned about the running of NHS dentistry, the networking with both colleagues and the area team and being involved in the further development of my profession within the NHS.

Not so great bits The amount of paperwork generated.

Top tips You need to have spare time and be organised. A willingness to get on with people to effect change.

Box 3.18 British Dental Association, British Association for the Study of Community Dentistry (BASCD): Dr Steve Boyle

What qualifications did you need for this role? For BDA roles, it is usually a volunteer position. These were often, but not exclusively, from being on a relevant committee. This could be local section or CDS group. For the BASCD, it was similarly from being 'elected' on to the central committee.

What does the role entail? Apart from attending the various committees, it involved stepping up to carry out specific tasks and keeping members informed and hopefully motivated. A major piece of work on the audit working group involved surveying members, developing teaching tools, producing conferences, lecturing and seeking funding for projects.

Great bits Helping to shape future developments in dentistry. A chance to participate in new and novel developments. Networking with enthusiastic colleagues. Some 'medical tourism'.

Not so great bits Some of the tasks impinged on personal time a lot, but usually that was OK. Dealing with apathy and criticism from others that it was a 'jolly'.

Top Tips Get involved: it's your chance to shape things rather than just be reactive! Do it early before cynicism sets in! (I think Steve means before you get too weighted down – Ed.).

Box 3.19 Dental professional network chair: Mrs Janet Clarke MBE

What qualifications did you need for this job? Registered dentist is the only qualification, but you need to have respect of colleagues, excellent networks throughout dentistry, confidence, resilience, ability to influence and negotiate, public speaking, assimilation of lots of information quickly. I could go on and on…

What does the job entail? Networking, networking and more networking, to, in my view, bridge the gap between area team commissioners and contractors and the local profession. Ensuring both are working together on the same page, designing and agreeing strategic direction and implementing plans. Meeting national NHS England and Department of Health demands, such as Call for Action and Contract Reform engagement.

Great bits? Meeting people, talking to them, thinking strategically.

Not so great bits? Time constraints: I only have 6 hours a week, which is nowhere near enough.

Top tips Be prepared for things to take far longer than you ever imagined and keep positive. Be nice to everyone: you may need their support at some point.

Top Tip: Don't ask the question if you think you won't like the answer
                                                                    Janet Clarke

Box 3.20 President, British Association of Dental Therapists (BADT): Miss Bal Chana

What qualifications did you need for this job? Qualified dental therapist. Membership in the BADT.

What does the job entail? As president, I serve as the figurehead of the association leading the dental therapy profession. I represent the association on various boards, working closely with the Department of Health and the GDC.

Great bits? Networking and meeting fellow professionals. Leading the profession forward.

Not so great bits? The time I need to dedicate to this voluntary role.

Top tips Be passionate about your role as a dental therapist and want to drive the profession. Enjoy meeting people.

Box 3.21 Chairman: Professor Ken Eaton

What qualifications did you need for this role? No formal qualifications. The skills required are gained with practice over time. In my case, military training in leadership and person management helped.

What does the role entail? Leading the organisation concerned and being responsible for its actions. When chairing meetings: keeping proceedings to time, trying to ensure that all members of the committee or group are able to express their views and act, as far as possible, as a united team.

Great bits? Helping the group or organisation concerned to develop. Helping members of the group to develop and progress.

Not so great bits? Having to correct poorly written papers or minutes.

Top tips Listen to everyone and try to involve them. Be happy to make final decisions.

Career Highlight: Being selected as GDC Clinical Adviser

Shazad Malik

Regulation

The main regulator of the dental profession is the GDC, but the CQC also undertakes a regulatory role, as does the Health Ombudsman. These are statutory roles laid down in law. The GDC has a number of roles in which dental professionals are employed, including fitness-to-practice (F2P) panel members, educational inspectors who visit dental educational establishments, clinical advisers and clinical experts. The CQC also employs dental professionals to assist in inspections and advise the organisation.

Box 3.22 Fitness-to-practice (F2P) investigating panel member: Mrs Geraldine Birks

What qualifications did you need for this job? Dental registrant, if a dental member. No specific additional qualifications required. Evidence of career professional development.

Great bits? I have learnt so much about dental regulation and I enjoy the teamwork involved in the panel meetings.

Not so great bits? I am required to be very self-disciplined, to ensure adequate preparation time before meetings in London.

Top tips Prepare well by finding out as much beforehand as possible. Believe in yourself and your abilities.

What does the job entail? All Investigatory Committee (IC) members are expected to embrace and demonstrate the principles of fairness, equality and diversity, and to comply with both the GDC's code of conduct for statutory committee members and the seven principles of public life (the Nolan Principles). Members need to demonstrate the competencies set out in the competency framework. The role of an IC member is to:

- Work effectively with other IC members to make fair, appropriate, timely and consistent decisions about complaints made against dentists or DCPs.
- Prepare fully for meetings, to enable the efficient operation of the committee, applying the GDC's standards and other guidance.
- Make reasoned decisions about applications for adjournments, extensions to deadlines and the admissibility of documents.
- Develop and improve as an IC member and contribute to the development of others using the Development Review Process.
- Contribute to projects as required for the development of the IC, including new-member induction and consultation on proposed changes to internal process and documentation.

(Source: General Dental Council, 2014.)

Expert witness

Expert witnesses can be utilised by the GDC, individual patients or individual dental professionals. They will usually be instructed by a barrister. Regardless of who instructs you, your role is the same: to assist the court or the hearing (in the case of the GDC) in reaching its decision. You are independent of either party and produce your report on the facts of the case. Most expert witnesses are instructed for their clinical knowledge and expertise, but some may be called because of their skills in nonclinical dentistry (e.g. education).

Box 3.23 Expert witness (GDC): Mr Steve Brookes

What qualifications did you need for this job? No formal qualifications, but they do insist that you still work in practice to a degree.

What does the job entail? Receive instructions. Read through, ensuring that all the documents required are present. Provide a draft report for counsel and individual patient audits as required, usually within 6 weeks. This stage takes ~10 hours in simple cases but can be extended by 1–2 hours per additional patient report required. Conference with counsel in London, ~2 hours. Provide final report, ~4 hours extra. Attend hearing, usually for 3–4 days, to give evidence and support barrister in case.

Great bits? The detail and searching through the notes to confirm or deny the GDC allegations. Pulling it all together in one coherent report. The interaction with non-dental colleagues lets you see the bigger picture. Protecting the patients. You feel that you are giving something back.

Not so great bits? The vague details about time you have to cross out of your diary for hearings. For example, they may ask for 10 days, but when you get there you are only required for 3. Seeing that patients have been harmed, but being unable to bring the case before the hearing committee as it will not pass the balance-of-probabilities test. At times, you are not able to protect patients.

Top tips Be prepared to work long hours late into the night to produce a report on time, sometimes for no pay. Be very, very thorough in your fact-finding – it is very embarrassing to be shown up by the defence barrister. You are playing games on their home ground.

Top Tip: Make eye contact and have a decent handshake

Janet Clarke

Development/support

Mentor

As a mentor, you are as likely to benefit and gain personal development from the partnership as the mentee. Chapter 5 will look at mentoring as part of career development and the benefits of working with a mentor. Chapter 7 will include qualifications and training to become a mentor. Here I want to outline the benefits of being a mentor as a career development. Many dental professionals gain considerable benefits from being a mentor, whether formally or informally, paid or pro bono. My belief is that mentoring will grow in importance as we move to more meaningful continuing professional development and remediation.

Let's think about what a mentor does and the characteristics they need. What they do:

- Give clear feedback to help the mentee identify what they need to do.
- Push the mentee out of their comfort zone, but not beyond their limits.
- Be there with the mentee, acknowledging and motivating them, championing them, encouraging them to take new steps.
- Encourage the mentee to explore the possibilities by being curious.
- Support the mentee to do a current job more effectively, offer insight into potential career paths and support their motivation and ambition.
- Be willing to share access to networks and connections, or provide insights into personalities and relationships of potential value to the mentee.
- Offer knowledge and understanding of the structural, political and social field of the workplace – both the visible and invisible structures – such that the mentee is better able to be resourceful, influential and successful in that environment.
- Act as a teacher at some times and as a coach at others.
- Listen: to be listened to is a rare experience, and the impact of this can be immense. 'Receptive listening' is about paying attention to the speaker's words and everything that surrounds them.
- Be a 'role model'.

Clearly, a good mentor can be many different things to many different people. It's not that you have all the answers – it is your opinions, and your honest belief in your advice, that will lead to success. Trust between mentor and mentee acts as the glue that binds the relationship together: if the trust is missing, the relationship won't work.

Coach

A coach supports people to get what they want, without doing it for them or telling them what to do. The coaching conversation is an art, a science and a practice. Professional coaches refer to the person being coached as their client or coachee. Coaches use a range of interpersonal communications skills. They listen more than they talk; they get the coachee to process their thoughts and ideas; they are empathetic and trust the coachee to see possibilities and to have their own ideas, solutions and answers. Dental professionals can make great coaches, but it can be difficult at times not to advise your coachee or tell them what they should do. This is where training is so important. I have given some pointers on where you can go for training in Chapter 5 and for qualifications in Chapter 7.

> *Career Highlight: Becoming president of the British Association of Dental Therapists*
>
> Bal Chana

Dental journalism

Dental journalism covers topics and issues of relevance and importance to dental professionals. Journalists write news stories, features and editorials.

Many dentists become involved in dental journalism. They may write for specialist dental publications, house journals, the health pages of national or local newspapers or their own opinion Web sites. Blogging is a useful way of learning how to write interesting copy that others like to read. Bloggers write opinion pieces and articles and post them on a Web site – often their own, but it doesn't have to be. Blogging allows other people to add their comments to yours. It can be a great way to learn how to write for the Web, which is a different skill than writing hard copy.

A number of dentists take on the role of editor, which again varies from editor of a prestigious dental journal to editor of an in-house magazine. There is a forum for British editors – the British Dental Editors Forum (BDEF) – which acts to promote good practice and the discussion of issues of common interest amongst members. It also encourages young dental communicators and has provided awards.

Dental volunteer – overseas

Being a dental volunteer is a life-changing thing to do. You might volunteer for a few weeks, a few months or longer. Whatever the period, the benefits you will gain are almost immeasurable. I was privileged to work overseas for just a few weeks in 1985 and I still remember what an amazing experience it was. I spent 5 weeks working in Muheza, Tanzania at Teule Hospital, a missionary hospital. I set up a dental clinic, providing the first dental treatment at that hospital. I also visited outlying clinics and undertook a survey of dental disease visiting schools around Muheza (Figure 3.1). I was the 97th dentist on the dental register of Tanzania at that time – and I still have the registration certificate to prove it. I learnt so much about patient management and my practical skills took a giant leap forward. I also had the opportunity to undertake surgery and saw some dental pathology that I had previously only seen in textbooks. It's hard to describe the wealth of personal rewards I gained, but they include resourcefulness, humility, confidence and a deep professional satisfaction in being able to impact someone else's life in a good way. It was slightly disturbing gaining the title of Daktari amongst the locals – some of you may be able to remember a television serial with that name. Those of you who are too young, be grateful.

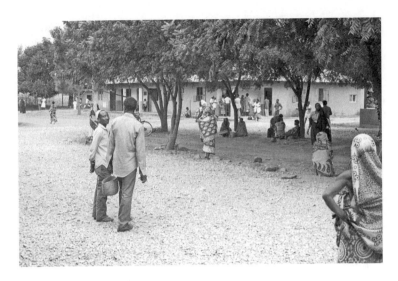

Figure 3.1 Teule Hospital, Muheza, Tanzania. November 1985.

Many dental professionals have discovered the satisfaction and benefits of being a volunteer. Here is an account from Dr Estelle Los, a GDP:

I had volunteered for various things all my life and happened to see an advertisement for the charity Bridge2Aid in a dental journal saying 'Dentists wanted for Tanzania'. Having spent nine years of my childhood in Tanzania I felt that this was a personal calling. My children had reached maturity and I felt the timing and relevance for me were right.

Volunteering as a dentist with Bridge2Aid involved joining a team of eleven like-minded, spirited, adventurous and caring people. We took out hundreds of painful teeth in people who had suffered for long periods of time whilst at the same time we trained six local Tanzanian Health Workers to do the extractions after we had left. The camaraderie was great, the patients were grateful and long suffering and the charity was very well run. It was one of the best experiences of my relatively well-travelled life, aged 54!

I gained friends for life, a direct understanding of the huge inequity in health care in the world, a sense of returning to my childhood homeland to give something back, greater confidence in my ability to deal with challenges both personally and professionally and a lot of extraction experience with no water or electricity and only a basic extraction kit.

I had been thinking of retiring from dentistry due to the increased burden of costs, CQC, litigation threats and demanding patients in the

UK but my experiences (I have been three times now) with Bridge2Aid turned me right around and I have no plans to give up the skills that can relieve so much pain in the world. I urge any dentist or dental nurse to get involved with such projects, what you have to gain is so much more than you give.

Both Estelle and I engaged in short-term volunteering, but there are opportunities to offer your expertise for longer periods. Dr Jane Davies-Slowik spent a year in Dharamsala, India in 1995. She shares her experiences here:

I had come to a crossroads in my personal life and had reached a point in my professional career where I felt I needed to take stock and decide which direction I wanted to take. I had always been interested in working abroad and felt that this was the time when I had 15 years' experience of work to be able to offer something more substantial. I had previously spent 10 days working in Israel as a volunteer dentist and was fascinated by being able to live and work with the people in that country, a very different experience to spending two or three weeks' holiday in a foreign country.

The description of the project resonated with my personal philosophy and values, and I knew when I spoke to other volunteers that this felt right for me.

If I hadn't done this I felt that I would have stagnated in the job I was in and I needed to take a step out of the 'rat race' and reevaluate my professional career.

I had one of the best years of my life working in Dharamsala, in Northern India with the Tibetan Government in Exile, training five dental therapists who would go back to their settlements in India and provide the only dental care within their communities. I worked with another British dentist, who became a firm friend. We worked closely alongside each other and had different strengths to bring to the project and needed to be resourceful with very limited equipment and access to information (pre-Internet). Our autoclave was a pressure cooker and we needed to wash our gloves between patients. Teaching these young Tibetans was so rewarding and it was fascinating to see what they could achieve with an intensive nine-month course ending up as safe practitioners. We arrived with the idea of practising ART (atraumatic restorative techniques) only to find that the local population was interested in being provided with crowns, bridges and dentures. The children were the most stoical, there was no provision of Inhalation Sedation or General Anaesthetic so if they needed an extraction, we just had to get on with it. Most people in the small town knew us as the Western dentists, and the gratitude they showed to us was truly humbling.

I definitely feel that I gained more from this experience than I gave. It was a real privilege being a part of the community and experiencing the culture, and highlighted how easy it is to make assumptions about people based on preconceptions.

There was a great community of Western doctors and dentists with a similar philosophy of life and I personally made some lasting friendships which continue to this day.

Professionally, it allowed me to go back to the basics of dentistry and never to assume that I know what a patient wants and values. The experience highlighted the rewards of dental education and the benefits of working closely alongside a colleague, sharing expertise and learning from each other and of evaluating what was safe practice as we allowed our trainees to undertake progressively more treatment.

I had some excellent training before I went to India on communication and teaching techniques, lessons which apply as much here in the UK as in the developing world. Life was simple and being on the edge of the community meant that I could work without getting involved in the politics of the hospital and health service, which sometimes gets in the way when providing care for patients here in the UK.

My greatest memories are of seeing the sun set on the Himalayas and watching the mountains turn red every evening, apart from monsoon time. Some colleagues and the Tibetan dental therapists and I had an audience with the Dalai Lama, just nine of us in his house further up the mountain. It was an inspirational visit and the look of awe and respect on our students' faces was uplifting and unforgettable.

There are a number of dental charities that provide dental volunteers overseas. It you want more information about what is available and how much money you will need to raise, I have included some contact details at the end of the chapter. This list is not comprehensive and other charities and organisations also aid volunteering overseas. A good start is an Internet search for 'dental volunteers overseas'.

I like wild ducks, but I like them to fly in formation

Unknown

Dental historian

Historians study and write about history, usually publishing their research. Dental historians study dentistry, dental professionals and all things associated with dentistry. We have a rich history just waiting to be uncovered.

For most dental professionals, dental history is likely to be a passing interest, but a few find it so interesting and absorbing that they add it to their career portfolio. My own interest in dental history was piqued by one Dr John Henry Holiday, dentist and contemporary of Wyatt Earp. The Lindsay Society for the History of Dentistry is an excellent place to begin to widen your appreciation. Perhaps your interest will lead you to research and write articles. I have included information about the Society of Apothecaries, which provides a Diploma in the History of Medicine. The BDA Museum and the Royal College of Surgeons Hunterian Museum are also good places to visit. The Dental Institute at Kings College London appointed the first UK Professor of Dental History in 2010: Professor Stanley Gelbier.

The eagle-eyed amongst you will have noticed that I have not expanded on general management. It has been touched upon in a number of the role accounts given by colleagues and forms an essential part of many jobs. In Chapter 5, you will find a case study of Professor Ros Keeton, a chief executive. Her story and CV will be of considerable interest to those who are interested in following this career path.

Useful organisations

Association of Dental Administrators and Managers. 2 Wheatstone Court, Davy Way, Waterwells Business Park, Gloucester, GL2 2AQ. 01452 729522. www.adam-aspire.co.uk.

Bridge2Aid. Established in 2002. Offers volunteer opportunities in Tanzania. They have recently started a pilot programme in Rwanda. 0845 850 9877. www.bridge2aid.org.

British Association of Clinical Dental Technicians. 44–46 Wollaton Road, Beeston, Nottingham, NG9 2NR. www.bacdt.org.uk.

British Association of Dental Nurses. PO Box 4, Room 200, Hillhouse International Business Centre, Thornton-Cleveleys, Lancashire, FY5 4QD. 01253 338360. www.badn.org.uk.

British Dental Association. 64 Wimpole Street, London, W1G 8YS. 020 7935 0875. www.bda.org.

British Dental Editors Forum. www.bdef.org.uk.

British Society of Dental Hygiene and Therapy. 3 Kestrel Court, Waterwells Business Park, Waterwells Drive, Quedgley, Gloucester, GL2 2AT. 01452 886 365. enquiries@bsdht.org.uk. www.bsdht.org.uk.

Dentaid. Offers opportunities in Cambodia, Uganda, Zimbabwe, Kenya, Malawi and Romania. 07970 163 798. barbara@dentaid.org. www.dentaid.org.

Dental Technologists Association. 3 Kestrel Court, Waterwells Drive, Waterwells Business Park, Gloucester, GL2 2AT. 0870 243 0753. www.dta -uk.org.

Lindsay Society for the History of Dentistry. https://www.bda.org/museum /dental-links/lindsay-society.

National Association of Prison Dentistry UK. PO Box 32, Stroud, Gloucestershire, GD6 1DL. www.napduk.org.

Orthodontic National Group. 12 Bridewell Place, London, EC4V 6AP. www.orthodontic-ong.org.

Projects Abroad. Offers opportunities in Argentina, Bolivia, Cambodia, China, Ghana, India, Jamaica, Kenya, Mexico, Nepal, Peru, Sri Lanka, Tanzania and Tonga. Where possible, tailors placements to the volunteer's level of experience and interests. 01903 708 300. www.projects -abroad.co.uk

Society of Expert Witnesses. PO Box 345, Newmarket, Suffolk, CB8 7TU. www.sew.org.uk.

Bibliography

Burke, F.J.T., Main, J.R. and Freeman, R. (1997). The practice of dentistry: an assessment for premature retirement. *British Dental Journal*, **182**, 250–254.

COPDEND. (2012). The Dental Gold Guide Third Edition, June 2013: A Reference Guide for Postgraduate Dental Specialty Training in the UK. Available from: http://www.copdend.org//data/files/Dental%20Gold%20Guide/3rd%20Edition %20June%202013.pdf (last accessed 18 March 2015).

Faculty of Public Health of the Royal Colleges of Physicians of the United Kingdom. (2007). Public Health Training Curriculum 2007. Available from: http://www.gmc-uk.org/MASTER_PH_Curriculum_150109_01.pdf_30534236 .pdf (last accessed 18 March 2015).

Gale, E.N. (1998). Stress in dentistry. *New York State Dental Journal*, **64**, 30–34.

General Dental Council. (2013). Standards for the Dental Team. Available from: http://www.gdc-uk.org/gazette/pages/standards.aspx (last accessed 18 March 2015).

General Dental Council (2014). Investigating Committee Guidance Manual. Available from: https://www.gdc-uk.org/Aboutus/Thecouncil/committeedocs /ICGuidance.pdf (last accessed 18 March 2015).

Gorter, R., Albrecht, G., Hoogstraten, J. and Eijkman, M. (1998). Work place characteristics, work stress and burnout among Dutch dentists. *European Journal of Oral Science*, **106**, 999–1005.

Humphris, G. (1999). Improved working conditions and professional support will benefit young dentists. *British Dental Journal*, **186**, 25.

Information Centre for Health and Social Care. (2012a). Dental working hours – Scotland 2010–11 and 2011–12, experimental statistics. Available from: http://www.hscic.gov.uk/catalogue/PUB07923 (last accessed 18 March 2015).

Information Centre for Health and Social Care. (2012b). Dental earnings and expenses, Scotland – 2010–11. Available from: http://www.hscic.gov.uk/article /2021/Website-Search?productid=8871&q=+Dental+earnings+and+expenses %2c+Scotland+2010%2f11&sort=Relevance&size=10&page=1&area=both #top (last accessed 18 March 2015).

Kay, E. and Lowe, J. (2008). A survey of stress levels, self-perceived health and health-related behaviours of UK dental practitioners in 2005. *British Dental Journal*, **204**(E19), 1–10.

Kay, E. and Scarrott, D.M. (1997). A survey of dental professionals' health and well-being. *British Dental Journal*, **183**, 340–345.

Myers, H.L. and Myers, L.B. (2004). 'It's difficult being a dentist': stress and health in the general dental practitioner. *British Dental Journal*, **197**, 89–93.

NHS Commissioning Board. (2013). Securing Excellence in Commissioning NHS Dental Services. Available from: http://www.england.nhs.uk/wp-content/uploads /2013/02/commissioning-dental.pdf (last accessed 18 March 2015).

Newbury-Birch, D., Lowry, R.J. and Kamali, F. (2002). The changing patterns of drinking, illicit drug use, stress, anxiety and depression in dental students in a UK dental school: a longitudinal study. *British Dental Journal*, **192**, 646–649.

Scottish Government, Health and Social Care Integration Directorate. (2013). Statement of Dental Remuneration – Amendment No. 123 (July 2013). NHS:PCA (D) (2013) 1. Available from: http://www.sehd.scot.nhs.uk/pca/PCA2013(D)01 .pdf (last accessed 18 March 2015).

Willet, J. and Palmer, O.A. (2009). An investigation of the attitudes and fears of vocational dental practitioners in England and Wales in 2007. *Primary Dental Care*, **16**, 103–110.

Chapter 4 **Coaching and mentoring**

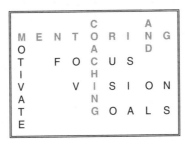

```
            C       A
M   E   N   T   O   R   I   N   G
O           A           D
T       F   O   C   U   S
I           H
V       V   I   S   I   O   N
A           N
T           G   O   A   L   S
E
```

> **Top Tip:** *You're not better than other people, but you are definitely as good as them*
>
> Janine Brooks

I am of the firm belief that all dental professionals can benefit from working with a mentor or a coach, and often both. Whether it be for personal development or career development, mentoring and coaching are invaluable. Mentoring for career development is extremely important. It can help you to discover career opportunities you did not know existed and it can help you explore those in which you are interested in more depth. Coaching, on the other hand, supports you to achieve your career goals. A coach can help you to clarify your ideas and think about what questions you need to ask.

There are two main aspects to this chapter: the importance of having a coach and a mentor during your career and information about what being a coach or a mentor involves. In addition, I have included sections on career planning, personal development and personal development plans (PDPs).

To begin, I'm going to describe how coaching and mentoring can help you throughout your career. Of the two, mentoring is probably better known and understood within health care and dentistry, so I'm going to start with coaching, just to be perverse.

How to Develop Your Career in Dentistry, First Edition. Janine Brooks.
© 2015 John Wiley & Sons, Ltd. Published 2015 by John Wiley & Sons, Ltd.

Coaching

Coaching has been shown to be a most successful way for people to develop their skills and careers *and* achieve their professional and personal goals. Behind every great professional, the chances are there's a great coach.

People at the top of today's successful organisations have a coach to help them to be the best they can be as individuals, to deliver personally and to grow their team. So, what's good enough for the likes of chief executives and managing directors is good enough for dental professionals. If you think coaching is just about sport, read on.

Jenny Rogers (2004) provides a simple definition of coaching 'that conceals its complexity':

> *The coach works with clients to achieve speedy, increased and sustained effectiveness in their lives and careers through focused learning. The coach's sole aim is to work with the client to achieve all of the client's potential – as defined by the client.*

The International Coach Federation (www.coachfederation.org) describes coaching as:

> *partnering with clients in a thought-provoking and creative process that inspires them to maximise their personal and professional potential. Professional coaches provide an ongoing partnership designed to help clients produce fulfilling results in their personal and professional lives. Coaches help people improve their performances and enhance the quality of their lives. [They] are trained to listen, to observe and to customise their approach to individual client needs. They seek to elicit solutions and strategies from the client; they believe the client is naturally creative and resourceful. The coach's job is to provide support to enhance the skills, resources, and creativity that the client already has.*

The key words that I take from these descriptions are 'achievement', 'maximise', 'partnership' and 'support': these words underpin the ethos of coaching.

> *When you can't change the direction of the wind – adjust your sails*
> H. Jackson Brown Jr

What it can do for you?

A coach supports you in your desire to move on in your career, uncovering your personal strengths and interests and matching them to the marketplace, so that you successfully achieve your next step. Career coaching helps you to recognise the talents you have and how they can transfer to other career streams, allowing you to see your strengths and have the confidence to get what you really want from your career. Many dental professionals only see their clinical skills; they don't recognise the many other skills they have developed (e.g. communication, project management, negotiation and marketing, to name just a few). A coach can help you to tap in to these sometimes hidden talents.

Coaching conversations cover the things that motivate, influence and inspire us from all parts of our lives, not just the work environment. Sustainable benefits happen when we work on our skills and intelligence, as well as what motivates us. Coaching looks at our emotional experience and our intellectual life and uses these experiences as resources to support change. The coach pays attention to the whole person: their personal life, their career development and their professional and leadership responsibilities. This is important when thinking about extending your portfolio or changing career direction.

A coach's attitude to their client/coachee is nonjudgmental, caring and supportive of their situation and needs. They create an empathetic environment so that the dental professional being coached feels safe to discuss the issues that are of importance to them. The coaching conversation is a confidential one and dental professionals undertaking coaching can expect the same degree of confidentiality as they provide for their own patients. Coaches help individuals to achieve their goals. They do so by asking questions that identify the gap between what they intend to do and what they are actually doing. A coach holds their coachee responsible for taking their own actions, doing the work necessary to achieve their goals and finding focus. The coach can 'hold a mirror' to reflect and understand the impact the coachee has on others. Knowing this helps the coachee to influence and engage others much more successfully.

Coaching is supportive, but it's not soft. Coaching challenges you to dig deep within yourself to reflect on how you behave and what your aspirations really are. Sometimes this can feel uncomfortable as you begin to understand yourself and what motivates you better. A coach will challenge you to think about new ideas and perspectives and to focus on what you want to achieve and what success looks like for you. They will help you to see what resources you already have and to identify what else you need in order to be successful. A personal coach will allow you to identify your talents and strengths, as well as your development needs. All of these are vital when considering your career opportunities and choices. A coach works in support of you and totally for you.

When a dental professional works with a coach, the coach will encourage them to 'ponder questions' and may well recommend ideas they can try out in practice. Coaching is not a 'quick fix'; for it to be successful, the coachee must work hard, both during the coaching sessions and between them. The coach will help them identify and set clear development objectives and goals and to review these at intervals so they can see what is working and modify what is not.

Top Tip: *It's good to talk*

Bal Chana

What exactly will the coach do?

A coach will ask relevant, probing questions, at times in challenging ways; they will acknowledge your accomplishments and help you to do more. Coaching conversations are not friendly chats; they have purpose, and the coach provides focus, bringing you back to the intended outcomes of the conversation. Coaching is about the person being coached, not about the coach. So, the coach does not allow their own style, preferences or feelings to influence the coaching process.

As I wrote earlier, coaches are like mirrors in that they reflect back to you your thoughts, words and ideas so that you can see them more clearly. You have the knowledge; your coach will help you to tap into it and give you the support and confidence you need to move forward. Coaching works to empower people by facilitating self-directed learning.

A good coach will spend a considerable amount of time helping you to develop your 'vision': where you want to be, what you want to do. As the Spice Girls espoused all those years ago: 'what you want, what you really, really want'. Mapping out your vision can take some time, and it's important that it does. Many of us want to get on with something, but it is a waste of time and effort if that something is not what we really want. Particularly when thinking about career development or changing career focus, taking the time to be clear about your vision is hugely valuable.

What makes a great coach?

There are more than a few coaches out there and it's good to know what to look for when choosing one. A great coach should be able to demonstrate:

- An understanding of today's demanding dental environment (although they do not need to be a dental professional).
- The quality of their coach training, coaching experience and qualifications.
- Their own leadership experience.
- Their fit with you.
- A positive rapport with you.

A great coach does not have to be a dental professional, but they do need to have an understanding of the environment you work in. However, the skills of coaching are different from the skills of being a dental professional and often it can be a bonus that they are not a dental professional, as they can bring fresh insights that we either don't have or have lost because we are immersed within our profession. We may not be able to see the wood for the trees.

> *Coaching is the art of facilitating the performance, learning and development of another.*
>
> W. Timothy Galway, *The Inner Game of Work*

> ***Top Tip***: *Enjoy yourself at work*
>
> Debbie White

What is the aim of career coaching?

Career coaching always focuses on moving forward from a foundation of the skills and experiences the client already has. It shines a light on the whole client, including their technical skills, transferable skills and personal skills. The process begins with supporting you to know yourself, then finding out about potential career opportunities, making decisions about those opportunities and finally constructing an action plan to move forward with confidence. A coach will work in support of you to achieve your goals. Career coaching adds the element of working alongside the client to signpost and open doors to opportunities. Aspects of mentoring and tempered advice can be introduced at this stage – but only with permission from the client.

Where can I find a coach for me?

Remember, a coach does not have to be a dental professional. Coaches understand people and how to get the best out of them. There are a number of dental coaches who work as sole traders, providing either face-to-face or telephone coaching. Not all provide career or development coaching, so check their Web site to see if this is part of their expertise. Some of the dental deaneries can link you to a trained coach, as can some of the specialty societies. I have listed some organisations that provide career coaching for dental professionals at the end of this chapter.

Having thought a bit about coaching and what it can offer someone who is looking for career support and development, I am now going to consider mentoring and what it can provide.

> ***Career Highlight:*** *Passing all my exams*
>
> Sophie Noske

Mentoring

Before going any further, it's important to understand that mentoring is about a relationship, rather than a process.

Mentoring means helping people to become better at helping themselves, helping them develop their opportunities and manage their problems, helping them become more effective, more functional, more empowered members of the workforce.

Nancy Redfern, Honorary Membership Secretary Association of Anaesthetists/Consultant Anaesthetist

Mentoring is increasingly being seen as a way of helping and supporting the development of people – in our case, dental professionals. The word 'mentor' has come to mean 'trusted adviser', 'friend', 'teacher' and 'wise person'. In dentistry, we are beginning to appreciate the benefits of mentoring, and increasing number of dental professionals are undertaking training to become mentors. In 1998, the Standing Conference on Postgraduate Medical and Dental Education (SCOPME) described mentoring as:

The process whereby an experienced, highly regarded, empathic person (the mentor) guides another individual (the mentee) in the development and re-examination of their own ideas, learning, and personal and professional development. The mentor who often, but not necessarily, works in the same organisation or field as the mentee, achieves this by listening and talking in confidence to the mentee.

I like this description because it includes the concept of guiding another in their own development and reexamination of themselves.

Two other definitions of mentoring also include concepts of support and development, which are essential aspects of career development and career management:

Mentoring is a supportive learning relationship between a caring individual who shares knowledge, experience, and wisdom with another individual who is ready and willing to both develop leadership qualities and partnership skills, as well as to realize a vision benefit from this exchange. The benefits received are professional career path growth and enrichment.

Adapted from Faure (2000)

Mentoring is a developmental relationship where one person, typically older, or more experienced, or with more expert technical knowledge, willingly and freely shares their knowledge, skills, information and perspective to support the personal and professional growth of someone else. In some cases the mentor may also share their contacts or networks.

The Forton Group (2013)

Mentoring can be a fruitful partnership at all stages of a dental professional's career, from the early days to preparation for retirement. Since the 1990s, it has slowly been gaining a position of acceptance and value within dentistry, with more and more dental professionals becoming familiar with the term and the concept. However, as Clutterbuck (2001) said, there is considerable confusion over what mentoring is and what it is not. It can often be confused with other methods of professional support. Counsellors tend to work with clinical issues and to go back to the past before going forward. It's often a one-way relationship. The key difference between the teacher and the mentor is that the teacher gives information; they know what needs to be taught and they tell their student what they need to know. A mentor has experience and will share it with the mentee; they are experts in their field. By contrast, a coach is often not an expert or specialist in the field in which their coachee operates. They ask probing questions to draw out solutions and clarity.

Mentoring is about wanting more just because more is possible. Mentoring focuses on the present and on the mentee's future desired outcomes. The mentor supports the mentee to achieve those outcomes, through a reflective, conversational process.

> **Top Tip:** *Remember, you are worth it*
>
> Sophia Noske

Beginning a mentoring relationship – being a mentee

If the relationship is to be of maximum benefit, you need to find the right mentor for you. Mentoring is not typically a partnership of equals and managing the power relationship issue is important for success. However, coming from a mindset of equal partnership can be effective in growing rapport. Good rapport between the mentor and mentee is very important; without it, trust can be difficult to establish. It can be helpful to create a mentoring 'contract' to manage expectations for both partners, covering the type of support and level of advice that the mentor is willing to give and the role(s) that the mentee expects the mentor to play. When establishing personal and professional boundaries, think about a code of ethics that will underpin the partnership. Confirm the mentee's objectives and goals, including potential and future roles, networks and relationships and their professional development requirements.

Managing expectations around roles and responsibilities is also important to the mentoring partnership. This will include setting a clear expectation that the mentee is responsible for creating their own results. Starting, maintaining and closing the relationship professionally will often depend on the needs of the mentee – on their goals and how quickly they wish to progress. To be successful, these will need to be matched with how much the mentor is able to give to the partnership. A mismatch can lead to failure. The duration of the partnership will vary. It might be focused on a specific goal or might be more related to professional and continuing development, becoming a more ongoing relationship.

When choosing a mentor, the power relationship between mentor and mentee should not be too close. What I mean here is that the mentor should not be the mentee's line manager. So, the practice principal may not be the right choice for an associate. A mentor who is more than two levels above the mentee usually constitutes too great a power distance, with which the mentee may feel uncomfortable. The compatibility of the relationship (between the needs of the mentee and the experience of the mentor) is of great importance. Getting on 'like a house on fire' is not necessarily effective in the longer term. The mentor must match the harmony of compatibility with an ability to address the mentee's needs.

Establishing a relationship is crucial – especially as the aim is to build a productive and equitable mentor/mentee relationship. The power of any working relationship lies not just in the strengths of each individual, but also in the link itself – and that link depends on equal input from both sides. A high degree of trust, openness and mutual regard is vital to a strong link.

Mentoring can take place through a number of different interactions, including face-to-face, by telephone and by email. Most mentoring relationships will utilise all of these. One consideration is how often the mentor and mentee should meet: this will depend on how much time each is able to devote to mentoring, the needs of the mentor and the objective of the mentoring. It is helpful to have a mutual agreement on all of this before the mentoring partnership begins. I would suggest negotiating a formal written agreement to reduce any misunderstanding.

What makes a great mentor?

- Someone who is experienced in the career aspect in which you are interested.
- Someone with wide personal networks.
- Someone who has the time to mentor you; however, if they have too much time then perhaps they are not very active in the field and they might be out of date.
- Someone you respect and trust.
- Someone who understands the role of a mentor; they will have acted as a mentor before and might have a qualification or training in mentoring.
- Someone in a good power relationship to the mentee.
- Someone who is honest in their opinions.
- Someone motivational.
- Someone who is open and willing to share their own successes and failures.
- Someone who is a receptive listener.

> **Top Tip:** *Adopt, adapt and improve*
>
> Derek Richards

The context of mentoring

A mentor often takes on many roles, as summarised in a model developed by the Forton Group (Figure 4.1). Roles include teacher, mentor and coach (hopefully not the fool).

The 'ask and know' quadrant represents the 'pure' mentoring context. The mentor asks what the mentee needs, knows the response that will help the mentee and is willing to share to support the mentee in moving forward.

The 'ask and don't know/don't need to know' quadrant is where the mentor takes on the characteristics of a coach. The coach asks great questions to which they do not know the answer – nor do they need to know. The role here is to support the coachee to discover their own answers from within.

The 'know and tell' quadrant is a place most people are comfortable in operating. Here the mentor acts as the teacher; they know information and are willing to tell their mentee.

If you find your mentoring relationship has entered the context of 'doesn't know and still prepared to tell', you should give serious consideration to ending the relationship. Your mentor has no experience of a situation but still gives you advice. In this context, everyone is having their time wasted.

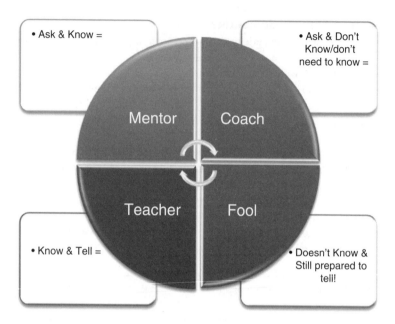

- Ask & Know =

- Ask & Don't
  Know/don't
  need to know =

Mentor   Coach

Teacher   Fool

- Know & Tell =

- Doesn't Know &
  Still prepared to
  tell!

Figure 4.1 The 'Forton Transformational Coaching 4-Quadrant Diagram'. Reproduced with permission of the Forton Group Ltd. (www.thefortongroup.com).

The challenge for a successful mentor/mentee relationship is in moving to the 'ask and know' and the 'ask and don't know' quadrants.

The mentoring partnership is orientated towards creating and possibility, not problem-solving: 'What do you want?' rather than 'What don't you want?' Taking the positive path rather than the negative path. It chooses conscious creation rather than simple reaction. The mentor brings their experience and knowledge to blend with that of the mentee in order to create something new.

Mentors should challenge the thinking of mentees, especially if they are stuck in one perspective. Mentors can offer ideas and advice. The perceptive mentor will notice shifts in the mentee's thinking, identify new perspectives opening up and offer new understanding of what is possible. Mentors need to keep asking questions and keep listening. The mentor should encourage the mentee to think differently. Options should be explored, drawing out the consequences.

Working with a mentor can help you to explore career possibilities and develop new insights into what you want from your career and the job opportunities that present themselves. A skilled mentor can support you to steer away from blind alleys; they can also help you unpick what is really important to you. Your mentor will be able to offer fresh insights, perhaps because they have dealt with similar situations in the past. Importantly, a mentor can help you to foresee difficulties and work through your approach to overcome barriers and obstacles.

I have had different mentors at different stages of my career – not always another doctor.

Professor Sheila Hollins, Past President, Royal College of Psychiatrists

This is an interesting quote, as it opens the door to working with different mentors and at different times. This seems totally logical: no one mentor will fulfil all your needs, and mentoring relationships will have a beginning, middle and a natural end.

Coaching and mentoring can be of help at any stage of your career, whether you are starting out, making a change or looking for new challenges. They are both 1 : 1 trusted relationships.

Top Tip: *Follow your dreams*

Bal Chana

What are the differences between a coach and a mentor?

Coaching differs from mentoring in that, put simply, a coach knows how to ask great questions so that the coachee can discover and learn for themselves, while a mentor knows how to answer great questions and pass on their experience. Mentoring is about giving experience, coaching is about finding experience from within. Coaches help you to use the experience you have gained and to really learn from it. They can help you to reflect deeply and to be your own teacher. A mentor gives you their experience, a coach uncovers yours. Great professionals have one or more mentor and one coach. Those are the high achievers.

Sometimes, we can get hung up on words and concepts. What is pure coaching? Is this pure mentoring? When are we advising? When are we teaching? An experienced supporter can use all these skills at the right time in the right place to give the help a person needs. Sometimes when coaching, I want to give a person a nugget of information (advise). When this happens, I always ask my coachee if they are happy for me to share my knowledge. I signpost that I'm moving from coach to adviser. I do that with knowledge and purpose: it's not accidental melding.

Mentors and coaches work with successful, healthy people and start in the present then go to the future. In both cases, a two-way relationship is established; for example, mentors and coaches will share personal information and experience. Both work by encouraging self-discovery and self-resolution.

A mentor is more likely to be an expert in the field and has been chosen because the mentee looks for advice and guidance from them. A coach does not necessarily have to have any subject knowledge in order to produce results. A consultant, by contrast, serves as an expert – a problem solver – who tells people how to solve a situation. Often, the consulting relationship is much shorter than the mentoring one.

Career Highlight: Being able to transfer skills and knowledge from dentistry to the wider aspects of health care and, thereby, build credibility for my profession

Ros Keeton

Where can I find a mentor for me?

Mentors tend to work within a professional domain they understand well and in which they have demonstrable skills and experience. You are likely to know an experienced dental professional who you would like to be mentored by. Some dental deaneries can link you to a trained mentor, as can the Faculty of Dental Practice (IUK) and some of the specialty societies. I have listed some organisations that provide mentoring for dental professionals at the end of this chapter.

Career planning

Chapter 3 covered many of the possible dental career aspects you might wish to pursue, but how do you work through what is right for you? This section on planning your career will help.

Career planning is the continuous process of:
- Thinking about your interests, values, skills and preferences.
- Exploring the life, work and learning options available to you.
- Ensuring that your work fits with your personal circumstances.
- Continuously fine-tuning your work and learning plans to help you manage the changes in your life and the world of work.

The career planning process has four major steps (Figure 4.2).

You can revisit and make use of the planning process all the way through your career whenever you want to think about making a change or enhancing your portfolio.

Start at the step that is most relevant for you now: the process does not automatically begin with thinking about your interests. It could be that your personal circumstances have changed and you want to explore new career options that fit these changed circumstances better.

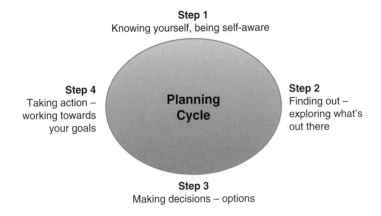

Figure 4.2 Steps in career planning.

Begin by thinking about where you are now, where you want to be and how you're going to get there. Once that is done, you can work on getting to know your skills, interests and values.

Step 1: Knowing yourself, being self-aware

Begin by asking yourself the following questions:

- Where am I now?
- Where do I want to be?
- What do I want out of a job or career?
- What do I like to do?
- What are my strengths?
- What is important to me?

At the end of this step, you will have a clearer idea of your work or learning goals and your individual preferences. At this step, a coach can be particularly helpful: this is where you set your vision for the future. You can use the information you gain about yourself as your personal 'wish list', against which you can compare all the information you gather in Step 2. Your personal preferences are very useful in helping you choose your best option at this point in time, which you can take further in Step 3.

Step 2: Finding out – exploring what's out there

This step is about exploring the varying aspects of dentistry that interest you. Once you have some idea of your preferences, you can research the specific skills and qualifications required for those new areas.

Explore roles that interest you and ask yourself:

- How do my skills and interests match up with these roles?
- Where are the gaps?

- What skills do I need?
- What options do I have for gaining these skills?
- Where is the work?

At the end of this step, you will have a list of preferred areas of dentistry and/or new role opportunities. This is where a mentor is most useful: they can give you helpful advice and open doors.

Step 3: Making decisions – options

This step involves comparing your options, narrowing down your choices and thinking about what suits you best at this point in time.

> **Top Tip:** *Be happy; it's contagious*
>
> Emma Worrell

Ask yourself:
- What are my best work/training/development options?
- How do they match with my skills, interests and values?

At this stage, either a coach or a mentor can help you hone the information you have gained and make choices.

Step 4: Taking action: working towards your goals

In this step, you have decided what option you are going to take and you are now ready to take it. This is the step in which you enrol in the course or programme you have chosen; you put in an application for a new job; you move forward. A coach can support you to make sure your actions actually happen.

Planning is an important activity and the discipline of logical thought is useful when considering the opportunities open to you. However, never allow a good plan to get in the way of serendipity. Many of the dental professionals featured in Chapter 5 have achieved the satisfying portfolio they enjoy through taking an opportunity when it arose and not being afraid to step outside the plan. A plan is a great thing to have and it will help your career development, but the plan is not your career. Use it, but don't be constrained by it.

> *You will fall over, but I'll be there to pick you up, brush you off and set you off again*
>
> Bob Izon

Personal development

The working environment has shifted from continuous employment to contracts, part-time working and greater movement between employers. There are no guarantees of either employment or career progression from employers. This means the individual is responsible for their own development and career progression. In dentistry, this is less of an issue than in many occupations. However, it does mean that each dental professional has to be able to identify their own development needs and identify the best way to meet them. We have to take responsibility and invest in ourselves, as it is very unlikely that employers or commissioners will do so. As registrants of the GDC, we are required to have a PDP, which I feel is essential for both day-to-day work and career planning.

Personal development plans

At its core, a PDP is a plan of what you intend to do over a period of time in order to develop yourself. As dental professionals, we must continually develop and improve ourselves if we are to put patient's interests first. Dentistry does not stand still; actually, very little does. If you, as a professional, do not have a plan for how you will develop then the chances are you are standing still (at best) or going backwards (at worst). Neither of these positions is good for you or your patients; if you don't work with patients then standing still is unlikely to be good for the business you are in.

A PDP does not have to be an elaborate affair: the basis is that you write down what you intend to do over a period of time, which is usually the next 12 months. However, like anything, it can only be of value if you put some time into it and really think about what development you need and want. As you will be aware, needs and wants are two different things. To give you a patient analogy that should seem familiar, patients may want aesthetic dentistry but actually need basic restorations and periodontal care. The want is far more attractive than the need. The same is true for personal development. You should look at both what you need and what you want and balance the two. For example, we all need to undertake core training in infection control, radiography, law and ethics, complaints management, emergencies and oral carcinoma, and these basic needs should be in your plan, if you have not met them already. Then you should add in what you want to do over the period; for example, you might want to gain a further qualification in an area of dentistry you enjoy and want to be even better in. Next, you should take a critical look at yourself and think about what you are a bit weak in and would like to strengthen. Finally, you should look at the basics of dentistry and whether you need to refresh and brush up on any of them. Don't forget nonclinical subjects as well as clinical ones. To summarise, in your 12-month plan, ensure you have:

- Core topics (try to do some each year – spread them evenly).
- Aspects of basic dentistry you need to refresh.
- Aspects of dentistry you want to develop.
- Aspects of dentistry you feel a bit weak on and need to strengthen.

Once you have thought about what you will include, you need to ensure your plan is SMART. That means what you plan to do is Specific, Measurable, Achievable and Relevant and you have a Timescale. Some examples are given in Tables 4.1 and 4.2, covering both needs (record keeping) and wants (endodontics).

While these two examples are for courses, your PDP can (and should) include other development activities. Table 4.3 lists a few for you to think about.

There are many ways in which you can personally develop; a good PDP has a mix of activities. A number of templates are available, either online or from your nearest deanery. However, it's not difficult to make your own template using the suggestions in this section.

> *The perfect is the enemy of the good*
>
> Voltaire

Table 4.1 Area for development: record keeping

Criterion	What it means	Example
Specific	Exactly what you will do	Attend a day course
Measurable	How you will know when you have done it	Course certificate
Achievable	Whether you can do what you want to do: Is it available to you given your budget and other resources? Do you have the time?	Yes, you can attend a local course: it is on a day that is convenient and you have no patients booked yet
Relevant	Whether it meets the need or want you have identified	Yes, you have looked at the learning outcomes and the course programme meets your need to refresh your record-keeping skills
Timescale	When you will do it – an actual date	15 December 2014

Table 4.2 Area for development: endodontics

Criterion	What it means	Example
Specific	Exactly what you will do	PG Dip Endodontics
Measurable	How you will know when you have done it	Satisfactory completion of course, award of a diploma
Achievable	Whether you can do what you want to do: Is it available to you given your budget and other resources? Do you have the time?	Yes, you can devote the time, you can cover the cost, your family and practice will support you
Relevant	Whether it meets the need or want you have identified	Yes, you lack confidence to undertake root canal therapy but would like to offer it to your patients
Timescale	When you will do it – an actual date	Enrol: January 2015 Complete: December 2018

Table 4.3 Nonacademic development activities

Activity	How it can help
Audit	Good to analyse outcomes and see where improvements can be made, e.g. record keeping, radiographs, consent procedures
Peer review	From another trusted colleague, you can learn different techniques and ways of conducting procedures
Case discussions	It can be helpful to dissect cases with colleagues and see what went well and what might need to be improved upon
Shadowing	Builds understanding of another role Helpful to watch someone more skilled in a particular area Useful for both clinical and nonclinical aspects of dentistry
Guidelines	Good to refresh new standards and underpinning knowledge Can form the basis of audits
Online resources	Can be particularly good for underpinning theory
Lead a project	Helps with leadership, team-building and organisational skills Helpful to learn about new areas
Reflective writing and logs	This should always be part of your PDP: you should reflect regularly on what goes well and what goes less well and on what learning you have completed: What did you actually learn? What will you do differently? Why?

Useful organisations

Providers of career coaching for dental professionals
Dental Coaching Academy. dentalcoachingacademy.co.uk.
Dental Deaneries. www.copdend.org.
A number of private dental career coaches can be found via the Internet.

Providers of mentoring for dental professionals
Health Associates. www.thehealthassociates.co.uk.
Dental Deaneries. www.copdend.org.
A number of private providers can be found via the Internet.

Bibliography

Clutterbuck, D. (2001). *Everyone Needs a Mentor*, 2nd edn. CIPD: London.

Faure, S. (2004). Introduction to mentoring: IM/IT community. No longer available online.

Honey, P. and Mumford, A. (1982). *Manual of Learning Styles*. Peter Honey: Oxford.

Rogers, J. (2004). *Coaching Skills – A Handbook*. Open University Press: Maidenhead.
Coaching

Claridge, M.-T. and Tony Lewis, T. (2005). *Coaching for Effective Learning: A Practical Guide for Teachers in Health and Social Care*. Radcliffe: London.

Connor, M. and Pokora, J. (2011). *Coaching and Mentoring at Work: Developing Effective Practice*. Open University Press: Maidenhead.

Jarvis, J. (2004). *Coaching and Buying Coaching Services*. Chartered Institute of Personnel and Development: London.

Rodgers, J. (2004). *Coaching Skills: A Handbook*. Open University Press: Maidenhead.
Mentoring

Connor, M. (2001). *Mentoring and Development Handbook*. Postgraduate Institute for Medicine and Dentistry, Northern Deanery.

Dean, A. (2002). *The Role of a Mentor for Newly-Appointed Consultants*. Royal College of Psychiatrists: London.

Egan, G. (1998). *The Skilled Helper: A Problem Management Approach to Helping*, 6th edn. Brooks Cole: Hampshire.

Forton Group (2008). Igniting Excellence in Leadership. Pamphlet. The Forton Group.

Forton Group (2013). Foundations in Mentoring: A Model and Resources for Mentoring. Pamphlet. The Forton Group.

Foster-Turner, J. (2006). *Coaching and Mentoring in Health and Social Care: The Essentials of Practice for Professionals and Organisations*. Radcliffe: London.

Garrett-Harris R. and Garvey R. (2005). *Towards a Framework for Mentoring in the NHS. Evaluation Report on Behalf of NHS*. Sheffield Hallam University.

Oxley, J. (2004). Mentoring for doctors: signposts to current practice for career grade doctors. Guidance from the Doctors' Forum. Department of Health Available from: http://webarchive.nationalarchives.gov.uk/20130107105354/http://www.dh.gov.uk/prod_consum_dh/groups/dh_digitalassets/@dh/@en/documents/digitalasset/dh_4089396.pdf (last accessed 18 March 2015).

Oxley J., Fleming, B., Golding, L. *et al.* (2003). Mentoring for doctors: enhancing the benefit. A working paper on behalf of the Doctors' Forum. Available from: http://www.academia.edu/1402110/Mentoring_for_doctors_enhancing_the_benefit (last accessed 18 March 2015).

Standing Committee on Postgraduate Medical and Dental Education. (1998). Supporting Doctors and Dentists at Work. An Enquiry into Mentoring. SCOPME: London.

Chapter 5 Case studies of dental professionals

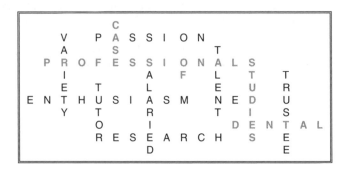

To paraphrase the words of a well known television advert:

The weather does lots of different things and so do dentists.

> **Top Tip:** *You can do it*
>
> Janine Brooks

I think the point is that dentists actually *do* do lots of different things. To illustrate this point, I've included in this chapter a number of case studies of dental professionals, which show something about their lives, their passion for dentistry, what they do and how they do it. After each dental story, I have added a potted curriculum vitae so you can see each person's dental progress. I am indebted to these generous fellow professionals.

> **Career Highlight:** *Setting up my own business(es)*
>
> Janine Brooks

I'll begin with me and my dental story: Janine Brooks MBE. I was born in 1956 in Solihull, Warwickshire, the middle child of three. I disliked school

---

How to Develop Your Career in Dentistry, First Edition. Janine Brooks.
© 2015 John Wiley & Sons, Ltd. Published 2015 by John Wiley & Sons, Ltd.

and left Tudor Grange Grammar School for Girls at 16 years of age to begin a life of work. I started at Aston University, as a junior technician on their technician training programme, one of ten trainees. I also began day release and night school and qualified with an Ordinary National Certificate, Medical Laboratory Technology and a Higher National Certificate, Haematology. Later, I used those qualifications as entry to Birmingham Dental School – not the traditional route, although I was not alone as a mature student with non-traditional entry qualifications that year. I qualified in 1983 and began work as a clinical dental officer in the Community Dental Service (CDS) in Herefordshire, and fell on my feet. The head of the service proved to be an excellent mentor, who helped to guide my career in the early years. In a few years, I took a chance and started to work half time for South Warwickshire Primary Care Trust in addition to Herefordshire, managing both CDSs. Reorganisation brought the opportunity to work full time in South Warwickshire and to take on general management responsibilities, so I started to manage a community hospital alongside the community nurses and health visitors, while managing the CDS and still keeping a small clinical commitment. After a while, I also took on managing a rehabilitation hospital, the learning disability team and the professions allied to medicine. Another reorganisation and a change of chief executive gave me the opportunity to take on project management of Y2K (not my finest hour – no problems and I missed out on the celebrations!) and the management of our merger with primary care groups, data protection and Caldicott Guardian duties. A while later, I began to feel dissatisfied: I felt I was no longer learning, just doing. This led me to take a part-time role as Caldicott Guardian with the NHS Information Authority (NHSIA), and I dropped some responsibilities in South Warwickshire. A year later, I heard about a new job with the National Clinical Assessment Service (NCAS) as part-time dental adviser. I took the leap out of clinical work, left South Warwickshire and worked across NHSIA and NCAS. The first arm's-length body review abolished the NHSIA and I was made redundant: a novel experience. NCAS became part of the National Patient Safety Agency and I was offered a full-time post as associate director (dentistry) for NCAS, and I took it. I loved setting up the dental service and working strategically with key national organisations. In 2006, I was appointed as an educational inspector for the GDC, and I have thoroughly enjoyed visiting educational establishments as part of the quality assurance of dental education since that time. The second arm's-length review in 2010 reduced NCAS's income by 25% and my department and I were made redundant: not so novel, but far more hurtful. I left in 2011 and haven't looked back. I'm now employed half the week for two different organisations: Health Education Thames Valley and Wessex and CDS CIC, a social enterprise (a nonexecutive role). The rest of the week, I work as a sole trader (Dentalia), travelling all over the United Kingdom for a variety

Dental Career Pathway	1984 Herefordshire CDS Community Dental Officer
	1985 Hereford–Muheza link, Tanzania Volunteer
	1986 Herefordshire CDS Senior Dental Officer
	1988 Herefordshire CDS Dental Services Manager
	1995 South Warwickshire Dental Services Manager
	1998 South Warwickshire Data Protection Manager
	2003 NCAS Dental Adviser
	2005 NCAS Associate Director
	2006 GDC Educational Inspector
	2011 Oxford & Wessex Associate Postgraduate Dean
	2012 Nonexecutive Director, CDS CIC social enterprise
	2013 Health Associates Founding Associate
Management Career	1996 South Warwickshire General Manager
Educational Career	1985 Herefordshire Dental Nurse Tutor/Course Organizer NEBDN Examiner
	1996 Northampton College Assessor (Dental Nurses)
	1997 Northampton College Internal Verifier (Dental Nurses)
	1998 City & Guilds External Verifier
	1998 University of Northampton Lecturer (Dental Nursing)
	2006 General Dental Council Educational Inspector (Quality Assurance)
	2011 University of Northampton Visiting Fellow (Dental Education)
	2011 Dentalia Coaching & Training Consultancy CEO Sole Trader
	2012 The Health Associates Founder
	2012 Dental Coaching Academy Founder
	2012 University of Northampton Senior Lecturer (Dental Nursing)
	2011 University of Bristol BUOLD Lead Tutor (Law and Ethics)
	2012 Birmingham Dental School Lecturer (Ethics)
Non-Dental Career	1972 University of Aston Laboratory Technician
	1974 East Birmingham Hospital Medical Laboratory Technician
	2002 NHS Information Authority Caldicott Guardian

Qualifications	**Dental**	**Non-Dental**
	BDS	Ordinary National Certificate
	DDPH.RCS	Higher National Certificate
	MCDH	NVQ Level 5 – Management
	Fellow FGDP(UK)	Assessor
		Internal Verifier (V1)
		External Verifier (V2)
		MSc Health Informatics
		Cert Med Ed
		Fellow Medical Leadership & Management Faculty
		Fellow Academy of Medical Educators
		Doctor Medical Ethics

Inspirational People along the Way	Barry Newey – Junior School Headmaster
	Bob Izon – Dental Manager
	Mike Marchment – Dental Manager
	Janet Clarke – Friend and Colleague
Interests	Family History
	Walking – Macchu Picchu Trail, Hadrians' Wall, Pembroke Coastal Path, Cornish Coastal Path, Thames Path, Great Glen
	Writing – my autobiography, short stories, flash fiction

Figure 5.1 Potted curriculum vitae: Janine Brooks MBE.

of organisations, providing training, and I personally coach a number of dental professionals. In 2012, I formed the Dental Coaching Academy with two non-dental colleagues. In 2014, we launched an online education centre to provide blended education for dental professionals in the United Kingdom and beyond. In addition, the Health Associates is a joint venture set up by myself and six other colleagues, not all of whom are dentists; we work together as and when opportunities arise. I have never been busier, nor more fulfilled. I love my career in dentistry and there is so much more I would like to achieve. So much to try, so little time!

> **Top Tip:** *If you don't ask, you don't get – so never be afraid to ask*
> Shazad Malik

Mrs Janet Clarke MBE

Janet is the clinical director of Birmingham Community Dental Service, one of the largest – if not the largest – in the country. She is a past president of the British Dental Association, chair of a Local Dental Professional Network and has wide general management experience.

She writes: I had a successful school career and decided on dentistry rather than medicine as I didn't fancy on-call. I enjoyed the undergraduate course: it suited my practical nature, plus my desire to get things done quickly. You can see I was achievement-orientated from an early age.

Community dentistry helped to consolidate my skills and to develop myself further, while general practice allowed me to prove to myself that I could hack it (I bought a Lotus Elan sportscar). I quickly did a masters degree and moved into a leadership role. I enjoy strategic thinking, and I am happy to work hard, with drive and commitment. These attributes are in short supply, so I found myself being given more and more responsibility, which I lapped up.

I got involved in local then national BDA roles, which met needs that my day job didn't and taught me lots. It also helped me to build a network of friends and colleagues. Even now, I am proud of my ability to work a room! My mantra has been to always say 'Yes, please' rather than 'No, thank you' (drilled into me by my paternal grandmother, who lived through rationing in the war), and while this has led me to sometimes being a tad overcommitted, it has meant I've had huge opportunities to develop and influence. Plus, I gain tremendous energy from this. Myers Briggs E, in case you hadn't guessed! I am a strategic thinker and influencer and not afraid to speak up. Leadership is in short supply, as is the ability to be decisive and confident. I think I can offer this and thrive on it!

Dental Career Pathway	1982 Dudley Dental Officer
	1983 Bartley Green GDP
	1985 Birmingham Dental Officer
	1988 Solihull Senior Dental Officer
	1991 Birmingham CDS Clinical Director
Management Career	From 1991 onwards, I have taken on increased responsibilities in the same post, so I have managed speech and language therapy, occupational therapy, podiatry and physiotherapy for a while. Medical director for a while. My geographical patch increased from South Birmingham to all Birmingham to Birmingham, Dudley, Sandwell and Walsall. My patch now includes Birmingham Dental Hospital, too
Non-Dental Career	As above, taking on additional responsibility through the years
Qualifications	**Dental** BDS, DDPH.RCS, MCDH, FDS Ad eundum **Non-Dental** Dip Health Services Management
Inspirational People along the way	Ros Hamburger, CDPH, for being so positive, but also so understanding of human frailty Sylvia Fry, my first management boss, for showing me how to file tedious things in a drawer, get them out in 6 months' time and throw them away Dame Margaret Seward for being fun, feminine and totally focused
Interests	Networking and friends Talking Politics and current affairs Family The sea

Figure 5.2 Potted curriculum vitae: Janet Clarke MBE.

> *Career Highlight: Successful negotiation of salaried dentists contract (87% in favour of national ballot – I can still taste the champagne)*
>
> Janet Clarke

Miss Bal Chana

Bal is a hygienist/therapist who began her dental career as a dental nurse. She is politically active and takes on a variety of educational roles, including educational inspector for the GDC. In 2014, she stepped down from a 4-year term as president of the British Association of Dental Therapists.

She writes: Towards the end of my schooling I had a strong desire to be a dental therapist. However, New Cross, the only school at that time, was due to close, so I decided to train as a dental nurse, which was a full-time college course that entailed going to various general dental practices for training. I worked for a number of years as a dental nurse, then as an instructor dental nurse (IDN). This involved teaching dental students close-support dentistry. I finally applied to the London Hospital, which was the new school to train dental therapists following the closure of New Cross. Eight students a year were selected to train; I was fortunate to be selected and achieved my ambition in life.

Upon qualifying in 1992, I worked in the CDS 3 days a week for 12 years, which I thoroughly enjoyed. This gave me the grounding to later join the world of teaching. I was fortunate to get this position as there were not many jobs for dental therapists at that time, due to restrictions on employment. As dental therapists, we could only work in the CDS and hospital services. This restriction was lifted in 2002 and dental therapists are now allowed to work in general dental practice. The other 2 days, I worked as a dental hygienist in a general dental practice, where I am still working to this day.

In 1998, I was appointed as a part-time tutor dental therapist at The Eastman Dental Hospital, where they were commencing a new dental therapy training programme. I worked there for a few years, and then moved to the London Hospital as a tutor hygienist and therapist. I was appointed as deputy principal dental hygiene and therapy tutor in 2004; this role I undertake for 3 days a week. In 2002, I also become a regional representative for the British Association of Dental Therapists; I held this position for 2 years and was then appointed as education and training officer. In 2006, I became the chair. At the end of my chair, I was ready to retire from the association, but I was asked to stay on and stand for president. I commenced my 4-year term as president in 2010. I am on a number of boards and committees, and am also a DCP inspector for the GDC, inspecting DCP training courses. I am proud to have led the proposal for direct access for dental therapists, which we finally gained in 2013. I was humbled to be the first recipient of the Dental Therapist of the Year award in 2006. There is not a day in my life that I feel I do not want to go to work. I enjoy teaching and get fulfilment from seeing my students succeed. I also love restorative care and, as funny as it may sound to some, I get excited by the sight of a dental drill. I take pride in trying to achieve perfection in the work that I do.

Dental Career Pathway	1983 National Certificate for Dental Surgery Assistants
	1985 Royal Society of Health Diploma in Dental Health Education
	1988 City and Guilds Further Education Teachers Certificate
	1992 Diploma in Dental Hygiene
	1992 Diploma in Dental Therapy
	2002 BADT London Regional Representative
	2004 BADT Education and Training Officer
	2006 BADT Chair
	2006 Royal College of Surgeons Dental Care Professionals Advisory Board
	2007 Dentsply How-To Guides
	2009 Working Group – Dental Skills Mix
	2010 Programme Planning Committee – BDA Conference 2011
	2010 BADT President
	2012 Games Maker – Dental Unit (Dental Hygienist and Therapist) at the
	2012 Olympics
	2013 Department of Health (DH) – Prevention Toolkit – Working Group
	2014 Dental Defence Union (DDU) Council Member, Committee Member,
	Dental Advisory Board Member
Educational Career	1998 Eastman Dental Hospital Tutor Dental Hygienist/Therapist
	2001 Barts and The London Tutor Dental Hygienist/Therapist
	2004 Deputy Principal Dental Hygiene and Therapy Tutor
	2006 General Dental Council DCP Inspector
	2007 Internal Examiner for Diploma in Dental Therapy
	2008 Royal College of Surgeons Assessor – Key Skills for DCPs
	2008 Liverpool Dental Hospital External Examiner
	2009 Cardiff Dental School External Examiner
	2009 Dentsply/Smile-On – Webinar – Periodontal Maintenance
	2009 DH Working Group on Dental Skill Mix
	2010 External Examiner Leeds Dental Hospital
	2010 Dentsply/Smile-On – Webinar – Manual versus Ultrasonic Instrumentation
	2012 Poster Presentation IADR Hong Kong
	2013 Direct Access Debate – The Dentistry Show
	2013 KL Malaysia – Training of the UK Dental Therapist International Speaker
	2014 Bristol Dental Hospital External Examiner
Qualifications	**Dental** **Non-Dental**
	Dip Dental Health Education Further Education Teachers Certificate
	Dip Dental Hygiene
	Dip Dental Therapy
Inspirational People along the Way	Dame Margaret Seward
Interests	Fine Dining
	Travel

Figure 5.3 Potted curriculum vitae: Bal Chana.

> **Top Tip:** *Work hard, play hard*
>
> Bal Chana

Dr Shazad Khan Malik

Shazad is a general dental practitioner who enjoys the diversity of being a foundation trainer and an educational inspector for the GDC and the politics of being a member of the LDC.

He writes: I was born in 1973 in Pakistan and came to the United Kingdom at 3 years old. Oddly enough, I still remember the flight! I am the oldest of my siblings, with two younger sisters and one brother. From a young age, I was always fascinated with biology. Initially, I had my heart set on being a medical doctor. However, I just missed out on my grades for medical school. So I decided to completely change career after listening to my cousin, who is a chemical engineer. I applied to Imperial College for Chemical Engineering and got accepted. After 3 months, I realised fluid mechanics and thermodynamics weren't for me. My mother suggested dentistry – at the time, I remember saying I would never look down into people's mouths for the rest of my life. Famous last words; never say never. Thinking I would get into medicine via dentistry, I applied and started enjoying dentistry and have never looked back. I did my Foundation Training in East London and thoroughly enjoyed it, and decided to stay in general practice. I enjoyed my Foundation Training year and at the time thought I would go on to become a Foundation Trainer one day. I very much wanted to get involved with dentistry at a local level, and in 2004 applied to be an LDC member. I bought into my own practice in 2005 and finally, in 2007, I became a Foundation Dentist Trainer. I then felt I needed to better understand my Foundation Trainee, so decided to do a Postgraduate Certificate in Medical & Dental Education. I would strongly encourage my Foundation Dentist to do their Membership of Royal College of Surgeons exam. I then decided to do the exam myself in 2009 and completed it in 2010. This was a proud moment for me. Being involved with Foundation Training, I felt it would be a natural progression to look at undergraduate dental education. In 2012, I applied to become a GDC inspector for quality assurance and felt very privileged to be selected. At the same time, I applied and was selected to be a Good Practice Scheme assessor: again, a very proud moment. Finally, in 2014, I applied and again was selected to be a GDC clinical advisor.

> **Career Highlight:** *My first job*
>
> Janine Brooks

Pre-Dental career	Fosters Clothing Company Part Sales Assistant
Dental Career Pathway	1998 BDS (Lond) Bart's & The Royal London Medical College, Queen Mary University of London
	1998 Foundation Dentist
	1999 Associate Dentist
	2004 Local Dental Committee Member
	2005 Principal Dentist
	2009 Waltham Forest PCT Subcommittee for Clinical Governance
	2010 BDA Forest Section Secretary
	2012 BDA Good Practice Assessor
Educational Career	2007 (to present) Foundation Dentist Trainer
	2012 General Dental Council Education Inspector (Quality Assurance)
	2014 General Dental Council Clinical Advisor
Non-Dental Career	2006–2010 Parent Governor

Qualifications	**Dental**	**Non-Dental**
	BDS	Fellow Higher Education Academy
	MFDS RCSEd	
	Pg. Cert Medical & Dental Education	
	Pg. Cert Dental Law & Ethics	

Inspirational People along the Way	My Mother and Father
	Dr Mohammed Khalid Mushtaq – Friend and Colleague
	Mr Edward Doff – Foundation Trainer
	Mr Raj Rattan – Associate Dean London Deanery
Interests	Reading
	Travel (when I get time)

Figure 5.4 Potted curriculum vitae: Shazad Khan Malik.

Dr Emma Worrell

Emma is a maxillofacial prosthetist and a visiting professor to the Princess Nora Bint Abdurrahman University Dental School in Saudi Arabia. She is an editor and published researcher with considerable management experience. Recently, she has been working on exciting new techniques for prosthetic eye replacement.

She writes: I am the classic late developer. I was only interested in hockey and sports at school. It wasn't until I could use both my manual dexterity/creativity (my father was an inventor, so it's in the genes) and science interests together that I became even vaguely interested in anything academic. Since I discovered the field of maxillofacial prosthetics, I haven't stopped treating patients, learning and being innovative in aiding the treatment of my patients. I manage to encompass both clinical and research aspects within my NHS job. I love my job and wouldn't know what I'd do if I didn't do this. Additionally, I mentor students here in the United Kingdom

Dental Career Pathway	1985 Guy's Hospital Maxillofacial/Prosthetic Technician
	1991 The Royal London Hospital Maxillofacial/Prosthetic Technician
	1992 Great Ormond Street Hospital for Children NHS Trust Consultant Maxillofacial Prosthetist
	1992 Institute of Child Health, University of London Honorary Research Fellow
	2010 Royal Alexandra Children's Hospital NHS Trust, Royal Sussex County Hospital Consultant Maxillofacial Prosthetist
	2011 Maxillofacial & Orthodontic Laboratory, Queen Victoria Hospital Maxillofacial Prosthetist
	Chief investigator in numerous random controlled trials
	Deputy editor for two publications:
	• *The Journal of Maxillofacial Prosthetics & Technology*
	• *World Coalition of Anaplastologists*
	Paper reviewer for:
	• *Ophthalmic Plastic and Reconstructive Surgery*
	• *The Eye and Opthalmology*
	• *British Journal of Ophthalmology*
	• *The Journal of Maxillofacial Prosthetics & Technology*
	• *Cleft Palate Craniofacial Journal*
	Collated and co-edited two maxillofacial publications:
	• *Prosthetic Rehabilitation of the Facial and Bodily Disfigured Patient* by Keith F. Thomas. Quintessence Publishing, 1994
	• *The Art of Clinical Anaplastology – Introducing a New Textbook Specifically Dealing with Facial and Somato Prostheses* by Keith F. Thomas. Self-published by K. Thomas, 2007
Management Career	1992 Great Ormond Street Hospital and North Thames East Cleft Centre, St. Andrew's Centre Maxillofacial & Dental Laboratory Manager
	2001 Great Ormond Street Hospital Performance Reviews & Development Plans
	2010 Royal Alexandra Children's Hospital NHS Trust, Royal Sussex County Hospital Maxillofacial & Dental Laboratory Manager
Educational Career	2013 Princess Nora Bint Abdurrahma University, Saudi Arabia Visiting Professor
	2010 HEE Thames Valley & Wessex External Lecturer
Non-Dental Career	2005 ABBE Level 4 Diploma in Home Inspection

Qualifications	**Dental**	**Non-Dental**
	BTEC, HNC, PhD	GCP, ECDL, ABBE Level 4 Diploma in Home Inspection

Inspirational People along the Way	Dr Michael Mars –Lead Consultant Orthodontist to the North Thames Cleft Lip and Palate Centre, Great Ormond Street Hospital for Children. He was founder and Chairman of Trustees of CLAPA (Cleft Lip and Palate Association). He nurtured me, supervised me academically and taught me to always have faith in myself – very much the 'can do' attitude that has changed my life pathway
Interests	Travelling with work and for pleasure
	Walking with my dogs

Figure 5.5 Potted curriculum vitae: Emma Worrell.

(MSc and Scientist Training Programme (STPs)) and I am a visiting professor in Saudi Arabia. I love the variety of my day job and enjoy the busyness of all my academic nuances. I hope to inspire the next generation to think laterally, not just treat patients in the same old way; to read current research, reflect on current practice and challenge how things are done; and to create a climate of writing and practising evidence-based/best practice.

> **Top Tip:** *Try to vary your work*
>
> Shazad Malik

Mrs Sophie Noske

Sophie is an orthodontic therapist who began her dental career as a dental nurse. She is also an examiner for the Royal College of Surgeons.

She writes: I was born in Epsom in 1976. My mum is English and my dad Canadian. I am the youngest of two: my sister Juliette is 2 years older than me. After leaving school in 1993, I went to Equine College for 2 years. I then went to the United States in the summer of 1995 to do Camp America. Coming back, I really wanted to start some kind of career and went looking for a job. I found a dental nurse job and that's where it all began. I studied for my dental nursing qualification and got hungry for study. I have enjoyed completing various courses and exams, along the way working in various practices from general dental to specialist (implantology, periodontics, endodontics and orthodontics). I was so happy when all my qualifications came together as a diploma in dental nursing. The same year, I started orthodontic therapy. I always worked full time until 2 years ago when I had my son; I now work part time and continue to examine on the RCS (Eng) OT exam. I qualified as an orthodontic therapist in 2008 from the Yorkshire Orthodontic Therapy Course after receiving a City & Guilds Diploma in Dental Nursing in 2007. Previously, I was a qualified dental nurse for 12 years, and in that time I completed post-registration courses in dental radiography, oral health education and orthodontic nursing. I am an examiner for the Orthodontic Therapy Examination at the Royal College of Surgeons in England and a member of the Orthodontic Nurses and Therapists National Group. Continuing professional development is important to me and I attend courses with the British Orthodontic Society and other teaching bodies.

I enjoy helping others achieve their goals and mentoring. I also like spending time with my family and cooking.

Because orthodontic therapy is quite a new addition to the family of dental professionals, I asked Sophie if she would write a little about gaining the orthodontic therapy qualification. She kindly agreed (see Box 5.1).

Pre-Dental career	Brinsbury College of Agriculture and Horticulture – Equine Studies – riding and stable management, levels 1 & 2 and Preliminary Instructor
Dental Career Pathway	1996 Started Dental Nursing 1999 Orthodontic Nurse 2001 Specialist Dental Nurse (Periodontology, Implantology) 2004 Specialist Orthodontic Nurse 2007 Orthodontic Therapist 2013 Orthodontic Therapist Practice Trainer
Educational Career	2008 Student Mentor 2009 First year of South Wales Course OT 2009 Fellow Colleague on Warwick University OT Course 2010 Examiner for Royal College of Surgeons of England
Qualifications	**Dental** National Certificate in Dental Nursing Certificate in Dental Radiography Certificate in Oral Health Education Orthodontic Nursing LCGI Diploma in Dental Nursing Diploma in Orthodontic Therapy
Inspirational People along the Way	Mrs Wakely – Form Tutor in High School Christine Gill – Best Friend Roshan Fernandez – Friend and Dentist James Stubbs – My Trainer for OT Simon Littlewood – Director of the Yorkshire OT Course
Interests	Walking Cooking Travel – Japan, Thailand, Canada etc.

Figure 5.6 Potted curriculum vitae: Sophie Nosk.

Box 5.1 Mrs Sophie Noske

What qualifications did you need for this job? National Examining Board for Dental Nurses (NEBDN) Certificate in Dental Nursing (it would be good if you also have experience in orthodontic nursing).

What does the job entail? Working closely alongside an orthodontist carrying out work under a prescription within our limitations. For example: placing, removing and adjusting fixed appliances; fitting retainer; preadjusted removable appliances; taking impressions; taking photographs.

Great bits? Seeing treatment from start to finish and how happy the patients are. Completing a difficult task well.

Not so great bits? Sometimes having to wait for the orthodontist to examine your patient and give a prescription before you can begin. They are often so busy with patients.

Top tips Go for it: it will change your life. Make sure you have a supportive trainer who respects your limitations.

Professor Ros Keeton

Ros is a dentist who moved into management and leadership within the NHS. She is currently the chief executive of Birmingham Women's Hospital. She is a great example of how dental professionals can impact positively on wider health care and how the skills we acquire in dentistry are highly portable and transferable. She retains close links with dentistry, both locally and nationally.

She writes: I was born in 1957 in Wellington, Shropshire, and grew up with my parents on the outskirts of London as a single child. I enjoyed school and always wanted to work in health care in some form.

I went straight from school to Liverpool University to study dentistry. I loved my time at university – I was not a serious student and spent most of my time enjoying the social aspects of living away from home! Once qualified, I went into the CDS as this seemed to fit both my values and interests, particularly in relation to people with special needs.

My first job gave me the most amazing freedom and I was able to carve out a unique role in which I focused my energies on dental patients with a broad range of special needs. I also became a member of the local Child Protection Team – probably one of the only teams in the country to have a dentist as a full-team member.

After 3 years, my husband, who was also a dentist, was buying his dental practice, so we left Liverpool and moved down to a large picturesque village in the West Midlands, where we both now live and where he still practices. As part of the 'moving deal', I initially worked half time for him in the practice and half time for Staffordshire CDS. I was never cut out to be a GDP, but saw my role as supporting him in his business. That role has continued, and although I no longer undertake any clinical work, I remain the clinical governance lead for the practice.

As soon as the practice was stabilised, I was lucky to have the opportunity to spend 2 days a week studying at Birmingham University for my Masters in Community Dental Health and a Diploma in Dental Public Health, Royal College of Surgeons. I found being a student for the second time around to be a very different experience, but I had the opportunity to work with Professor Andy Anderson (who I still have very fond memories of as an inspirational teacher and a lovely man).

As soon as I gained these qualifications, I applied for – and was successful in obtaining – one of the first senior dental officer roles in the country to combine an SDO position with some general management duties. This was my first step outside the comfortable world of clinical dentistry and something I really developed the taste for. Within 6 months, my general management portfolio had grown, and after 9 months I was appointed assistant unit general manager for community services. The senior nurse managers with whom

I worked in that role adopted me with passion and we had a huge amount of fun and success together. I stayed in North Warwickshire for many years, undertaking a variety of director roles, first as a chief operating officer and latterly focusing on clinical quality, which remains my passion today.

I finally left North Warwickshire, initially becoming a chief executive in Worcestershire. I did not have ambitions to be a chief executive – in fact, almost the opposite – but I was persuaded to apply for a 6-month post. The trust I inherited (a mental health, learning disability and substance misuse provider) was in trouble, and over the next 8 years I worked with my team to build a Trust I think we were truly proud of. The field of mental health was new to me, but this extension into yet another aspect of health care was something that kept me refreshed and interested. When the trust was dissolved to

Dental Career	1981 Cheshire Area Health Authority Clinical Dental Officer
	1984 Mid Staffordshire Health Authority Clinical Dental Officer
	1984 Partner in General Dental Practice, Kinver, West Midlands
	1988 North Warwickshire Health Authority Senior Dental Officer/Head of Community Services
Management Career	1989 North Warwickshire Health Authority Assistant Unit General Manager
	1993 North Warwickshire NHS Trust Director of Operations
	1999 North Warwickshire NHS Trust Research & Development Director/Clinical Governance Lead
	2002 North Warwickshire Primary Care Trust Director of Clinical Quality and Service Development
	2003 Worcestershire Mental Health Partnership NHS Trust Chief Executive
	2011 Clinical Commissioning Group Development, NHS West Midlands Project Director
	2011 Birmingham Women's Hospital NHS Foundation Trust Chief Executive
Educational Career	June 2013 Faculty of Health, Birmingham City University Visiting Professor,
	June 2014 Worcester University Fellow
Additional Career Information	2008 (to present) BDA Benevolent Fund Trustee/Honorary Treasurer
	An active member of the Central Counties Branch of the BDA for over 20 years, holding a number of roles, including president
Qualifications	BDS
	MCDH
	DDPH RCS
Inspirational People along the Way	Professor Andy Anderson – University of Birmingham
	Phil Jenkins – Dental Manager
	Lawrence Tennant – Chief Executive
Interests	Contemporary art and design
	Walking

Figure 5.7 Potted curriculum vitae: Ros Keeton.

form part of a larger organisation, I was not successful in gaining the new chief executive post, but moved instead to work for a very short time on a national leadership project and the development of Clinical Commissioning Groups. I found this a very different and almost abnormal job, as I was no longer connected to the front-line service or, most importantly, to patients.

I quickly moved on to become chief executive of Birmingham Women's NHS Foundation Trust, which again provided me with the opportunity to experience something new in a very specialist hospital offering both tertiary and quaternary services.

True to form, I have loved this new learning opportunity and engagement with a completely different group of patients. I love the NHS; in fact, I think I am like a stick of rock, with the words 'I LOVE THE NHS' written all the way through me. By far the best thing about the NHS is the people that work within it and what they give to the nation. My dental training and knowledge is the foundation upon which I have built my career. It has stood me in great stead and given me the credibility I need to undertake my many and varied leadership roles. I have had the opportunity to work with some fabulous people throughout my career, and I owe them and dentistry a huge debt.

Dr Derek Richards

Derek enjoys a wide and diverse career in dentistry. He has worked in the three major sectors: general practice, community dentistry and hospital dentistry. He is a senior lecturer, external examiner and consultant in dental public health. He is also well known as director of the Centre for Evidence-Based Dentistry and editor of the journal *Evidence-Based Dentistry*, as well as a Dental Elf blogger.

He writes: I was born in 1954, in Caerphilly, South Wales, the middle child of three. I had an uneventful journey through the school system; deciding what to do at university was my first big decision. Actually, dentistry was a spur-of-the-moment decision. At dental school, the environment was very sociable, and I took the role of year representative and was heavily involved in the annual charity pantomime. My first post in the CDS was a short but enjoyable experience, but general duties house jobs in Bristol beckoned, as did a hoped-for career in oral surgery. This was followed by oral surgery posts in Nottingham and Inverness (where I met my future wife). While oral surgery was much enjoyed, my attempts at primary fellowship were unsuccessful, so I moved into general practice. I realised that general practice was not for me, so I moved back to the CDS. A local bursary scheme provided funding for me to study for my Diploma in Dental Public Health (DDPH), which was the spur to returning to complete my fellowship. I now had the relevant qualifications to secure a training post in dental public health and I was fortunate to obtain a

post with Alan Lawrence and Sue Gregory. Shortly after beginning my training, I was introduced to Muir Gray, then regional director of public health,
and David Sackett, the new head of the Centre for Evidence-Based Medicine
in Oxford. This meeting was the beginning of my role in evidence-based dentistry (EBD). My specialist training was completed over 4 years, during which
period I undertook my diploma in evidence-based health care and was heavily involved in providing workshops and helping to develop and establish
the Centre for Evidence-Based Dentistry (CEBD) and the journal *Evidence-
Based Dentistry*.

Dental Career	1977 Cardiff BDS
	1978 Gwent CDS CDO
	1978 Bristol Dental School HO SHO
	1979 Nottingham General Hospital SHO
	1980 Raigmore Hospital, Inverness Registrar
	1982 Witney, Oxfordshire General Practice
	1986 Oxford Health Authority CDO, SDO
	1994 Anglia & Oxford Regional Health Authority Senior Registrar, Dental Public Health
	1998 Berkshire Health Authority Consultant/Director Centre for Evidence-Based Dentistry
	2002 Forth Valley Health Board Consultant/Director Centre for Evidence-Based Dentistry
	Editor, *Evidence-Based Dentistry*
	Dental Elf Blogger
Educational Career	1987 Oxford College of Further Education Dental Surgery Assistant (DSA) Course Lecturer
	1991 West Oxfordshire College DSA Course Lecturer
	1991 NEBDN Examiner
	1998 Oxford University, Evidence-based Health Care Tutor and Examiner
	2006 Glasgow Dental School Honorary Senior Lecturer
	2013 Dundee Dental School Honorary Senior Lecturer
	2013 City University London External Examiner Master Public Health Course
Qualifications	**Dental** **Non-Dental**
	BDS Evidence-Based Health Care Cert.
	DDPHRCS (U. Oxford)
	FDSRCS
	MSc (Dental Public Health)
	FDS (DPH)
Inspirational People along the Way	Muir Gray – Director of Knowledge for NHS
	Amanda Burls – Colleague and Friend
	Jan Clarkson - Colleague and Friend
Interests	Photography
	Gardening
	DIY

Figure 5.8 Potted curriculum vitae: Derek Richards.

After completing my specialist training, I succeeded Alan Lawrence as consultant in Berkshire. This was initially a part-time post, with some additional funding to help develop the CEBD, but it later became full time, and for a while I was covering Northamptonshire and providing some regional support with my colleague David Thomas in addition to CEBD activities. As a result of changes in the wake of the establishment of Primary Care Trusts, I became increasingly disenchanted with my role and position within the organisation. I therefore took the opportunity to apply for the part-time consultant post in Forth Valley. The part-time nature of the post provided me with an opportunity to devote some more time to EBD. However, I was then invited to become a specialist adviser to the Scottish Dental Clinical Effectiveness Programme and assist in its guideline development programme. More recently, I have again become a full-time consultant in dental public health, as we have developed a regional network to provide support to five Health Boards as NHS financial pressures have resulted in failure to replace retiring colleagues on a like-for-like basis. Recently, the CEBD has formally relocated to the Dental Health Services Research Unit at the University of Dundee, which is providing a number of new challenges and opportunities.

Professor Deborah White

Deborah White is professor of dental public health at the School of Dentistry, University of Birmingham. She is a well respected and widely published academic. She has undertaken a number of roles locally and nationally within the British Dental Association and is currently chair of the Central Committee for Dental Academic Staff.

She writes: I was born in 1954 in Bournville, Birmingham, the daughter of a marketing executive at Cadbury's, eldest of four children. I was educated at Bournville Junior School and then moved to Edgbaston High School for Girls, skipping a year in the transfer. I decided I wanted to do dentistry at the age of 14, having been to a careers talk at Aston University, and this determined my A-level choices, despite the fact that my O-level results indicated I should pursue arts subjects. I studied dentistry at Manchester University, starting at the age of 17, and was particularly interested in paediatric dentistry. I was part of the first cohort to experience outreach teaching in a community dental clinic, and this determined my career choice on graduation. I started work in Sandwell CDS in 1977, at first full time and then part time while I took up a part-time GDS associate role. I then successfully applied for a job at the industrial dental practice within Guest, Keen & Nettlefolds (GKN) and worked there for a year. This was an interesting role, treating everyone from the managing director to shop-floor workers. I then took about a year and a half out of dentistry to travel the world! We travelled overland to India and then hopped down through South East Asia, and I ended up working in a sandwich bar in Sydney for 3 months – an excellent life experience. When I returned, I got a job in the CDS in Walsall, and shortly after this had two children. I expressed a desire to progress my career and was fortunate to gain a place on the Masters in Community Dental Health programme at the University of Birmingham. I was then asked to undertake a part-time second-ment working on a major research project and I was hooked! A further two research projects followed, during which time I was exposed to the academic environment and some undergraduate teaching. In 1999, I decided to make the move from the CDS to an academic career, undertaking a PhD along the way. I then progressed to senior lecturer, became more involved in the edu-cation side of the role and became the director of learning and teaching, as

Dental Career	1976 Manchester BDS
	1977 Sandwell CDS CDO
	1978 Associate GDS
	1979 GKN Industrial Dentist
	1982 Walsall CDS CDO
	1987 Manor Hospital, Walsall Clinical Assistant in Orthodontics
	1991 Walsall CDS SDO
	1993 School of Dentistry, University of Birmingham Honorary Research Fellow
	1999 University of Birmingham Lecturer in Oral Health & Behavioural Science
	2000 Heart of Birmingham Teaching PCT Honorary SDO
	2002 South Birmingham PCT Honorary Associate Specialist
	2003 University of Birmingham Senior Lecturer in Dental Public Health
	2007 South Birmingham PCT Honorary Consultant
	2008 University of Birmingham Associate Professor
	2012 University of Birmingham Professor of Dental Public Health
Qualifications	1976 BDS Manchester
	1989 DDPH Royal College of Surgeons of England
	1991 MCDH University of Birmingham
	2000 PhD University of Birmingham
	2002 Postgraduate Certificate in Learning and Teaching in Higher Education
	2005 Fellow Higher Education Academy (FHEA)Registered Practitioner
Inspirational People along the Way	Professor Mike Lennon – University Lecturer
	Margaret Gray – Dental Manager
	Professor Andy Anderson – Research Supervisor
	Dr Gillian Bradnock – Head of Unit and Research Supervisor
Interests	Walking – I have completed the Coast to Coast path and recently walked part of the Northumberland Coastal Path
	Sewing – I am a member of a patchwork and quilting group
	Local Community – I am a member of our street association 'core group' – working towards improving 'neighbourliness'

Figure 5.9 Potted curriculum vitae: Deborah White.

well as carrying out epidemiological research (UK studies of child and adult dental health).

I progressed to associate professor, which is a learning and teaching route, and subsequently became a professor. I have a varied role as head of the dental public health research and teaching area, academic lead for paediatric dentistry, director of education and QA lead for the Dental Hygiene and Therapy programme, and until recently I undertook a clinical session in the CDS. I have had opportunities to act as an external examiner in a number of institutions and to visit dental schools in Europe as part of the Association of Dental Education in Europe. These experiences have enabled me to develop a broader understanding of the scope of dental education.

Dr Reena Patel

Reena is a dentist I met a few years ago who immediately struck me as someone to watch. She has drive and determination, and within a few years has experienced a broad spectrum of aspects of dentistry and health care that will be a solid foundation for her future.

She writes: I was born in Canada, and soon moved to Saudi Arabia, where I spent the first 10 years of my life. I had a fun childhood, dominated by bizarre memories of sandstorms and perpetual sunshine. I then spent the majority of my early 'formative' teenage years in Barry, South Wales. After a challenging transitional few months of settling into a new country and new culture (with an American accent), I started to really enjoy school: both academia and sport. We later moved to Surrey, where I completed my A-levels. Having decided that Wales was my chosen 'homeland', I returned to study dentistry there. Upon completion of my training, I was determined to start a new adventure, and upon securing a 2-year general professional training (GPT) post in London, I mapped out a stint of further postgraduate study, followed by a 6-month backpacking trip. I enjoyed GPT, and maximised opportunities to consider the various specialties of dentistry. Despite enjoying clinical work, in every post I was drawn to aspects of clinical prevention and efficiency in service delivery. However, I realised that, as a very junior dentist, I was not going to be able to gain further experience in either of these areas in the NHS unless I commenced a formal training post in dental public health, and I was not ready to do that yet. I felt that, at such an early stage in my career, with such little clinical and management experience, I had very little to offer. Driven by curiosity more than anything else, I decided to apply for an MSc in International Health Management. At the time, I felt that it would expose me to a world beyond dentistry, and would provide me with learning experiences that would help me to stand out within dentistry. Upon completion of the MSc,

I obtained a position at Deloitte, as a strategic management consultant. This was an extremely challenging career change, and I look back now and think I must have spent the whole time looking like a rabbit caught in the headlights. Everything was different: the working culture; competition between peers; a role not defined by professional standards. Given these differences, it was difficult starting such a position without colleagues in a similar situation. Most people starting out in a career in management consultancy enter at analyst level, through a graduate entry programme. As an 'experienced hire', you were expected to immediately walk the walk and talk the talk, despite coming from a very different background. However, I learnt quickly, and worked very hard, aligning myself with colleagues who were supportive and willing to give guidance and help. As the only dentist, I was able to carve out a niche for myself. However, as dentistry formed only a very small part of the overall NHS budget, this limited opportunities to be a specific 'dental' management consultant. With the general financial cuts to the NHS, I began to be used, more and more, as the token 'medic' on a variety of projects. Mindful that I was hired on the basis of a specific skill set of dentistry, I did not want to lose these skills and become a generic management consultant. I was concerned that I was losing my unique selling point so I decided to leave. This was not an easy decision to make, but I was later reassured by the fact that, within a few months, most of the other medics had left too. Deloitte simply did not have the insight to invest in developing their medical and dental experienced hires. I then commenced a post in the salaried services, an aspect of dentistry in which I had not previously worked. During that time, I was able to balance a clinical position with taking on individual pieces of commissioned work, in collaboration with Professor Kenneth Eaton. While this was challenging, I relished the opportunity to apply an academic and scientific approach in these projects, and was fortunate to work with a wide range of public and private-sector clients. The next 3 years went by very quickly, and I was then finally successful in securing a specialty training post in dental public health in the East of England Deanery. Looking back now, in my capacity as a specialty trainee, I can safely say that each role I have completed to date has provided me with extremely useful learning experiences and skill sets, which I regularly apply in my daily work. These are principally focused around project management, stakeholder engagement and developing written reports. I'm looking forward to continuing my training over the next few years and, for this little period, balancing babies and working life.

Career Highlight: Finishing my doctorate – only took 8 years!

Janine Brooks

Pre-Dental Career	Various waitressing jobs through university
Dental Career	2004 BDS
	2004 London Vocational Dental Practitioner
	2005 GKT General Professional Training, SHO Posts in Oral Medicine and Oral Surgery
	2006 Brighton OMFS SHO
	2007 Oversees Voluntary Work
	2010 Bromley Community Dental Services
	2012 Health Associates Associate
	2013 Specialty Training in Dental Public Health
Management Career	2009 Deloitte Strategic Management Consultant, Healthcare and Life Sciences Division
Qualifications	2004 BDS　　　　　　2008 MSc International Health
	2006 MFDS RCS　　　　　Management
	2014 MDPH
Quotes	'It doesn't need to be perfect – just good enough' Sandra White
Inspirational People along the Way	Professor Kenneth Eaton
	Sandra White
	Amanda Crosse
	Paul Batchelor
Interests	Travelling, pilates, cooking, swimming, competitive events: triathlons, half marathons

Figure 5.10 Potted curriculum vitae: Reena Patel.

Mrs Penny McWilliams

Penny is clinical director of primary care dental services with NHS Dumfries and Galloway. She is also a vocational training trainer.

She writes: On the advice of my then clinical director, in 1996 I started a part-time Masters in Public Health as an 'insurance policy'. When I had finished that, and because I still had back problems that reduced my ability to do clinical duties, I contacted Health Promotion in NHS Lanarkshire, where I knew the lead officer for oral health promotion, and started doing project and research work. The very different perspective that this gave me – moving away from treatment of individual patients towards consideration of group programmes – combined with the exposure to non-dental and nonclinical health care staff duly made me very much better equipped to apply for a dental managerial post, initially as an acting clinical dental director and then as a substantive appointment. I was very struck by the lack of former dental clinicians working in public health or health promotion, in comparison to former medical and nursing staff. I have become very aware of instances in which dentists and other clinicians are unhappy or uncomfortable within a clinical setting, for whatever reason. They tend to assume that their only options are either to move into dental education or to give up both dentistry and health care altogether. Often, they leave it very late (perhaps after extended periods of sick leave, due to stress) before considering diversifying or developing alternatives to their original clinical role.

I completed a part-time Open University Business School MBA. Since then, I have become involved in NHS Education Scotland (NES) Dental Foundation Year 2 Training as shared trainer, with occasional clinic cover duties for BDS Year Five Outreach dental undergraduates and undergraduate therapist Year 3 students in Dumfries.

Short biographies

I'm deeply indebted to those who have generously written their stories and allowed me to publish them for you. They are truly inspirational, one and all. Many other people kindly sent me their curriculum vitae/biographies, and I'm going to include some of those in this section so you can see the wide and varied careers dental professionals enjoy. The dental professionals you will read about here are all people I have met and who have struck me as enthusiastic, committed and deeply passionate about dentistry. The joy and the difficulty for me is that I have met so many incredible professionals, my whole book could be their profiles. My hope is that you will find inspiration to take your career further as a result of reading about these great role models.

Mr Ian Taylor

Profile Before focusing on crown and bridgework, Ian worked as a prosthetic and cobalt chrome technician for 4 years at Birmingham Dental School, between 1978 and 1982. His experience in partial chrome dentures, plates and precision attachments has held him in good stead when planning the challenges of complex combination cases for full arch or full mouth reconstructions.

Education 1989 City and Guilds Certificate Dental Technology

1990 Advanced City and Guilds – Crown and Bridge

2009–11 Advancement of Dentistry – achieved all five levels

2013 Clinical Dental Technician

Current Roles Castle Ceramics Dental Laboratory, Tamworth, Staffordshire. Employs nine GDC-registered technicians plus six lab assistants, providing a full service to their client base (formed 1986).

Career History In 1999, Ian and five fellow dental laboratory directors from around the United Kingdom formed the Private Prosthodontics Group (PPG). In 2011, Ian was elected by the Faculty of General Dental Practitioners (FGDP) to represent dental technicians on the DCP committee to help dental technicians develop their career and skill pathways.

Ms Margaret Nash

Profile Maggie is a dental nurse/DCP tutor involved in the design and delivery of continuing professional development events for DCPs, a higher education programme for dental nurses and the delivery of an established dental nurse post-registration course. She is a postgraduate student with an interest in research, in particular research that relates to and supports effective post-registration dental professional education.

Education 1982 NEBDN Examination for Dental Nurses

2007 NEBDN Certificate in Oral Health Education

2012 BSc (Hons) in Primary Dental Care, University of Kent

Current Roles General Dental Council Fitness to Practice, DCP member Freelance DCP Tutor (contracted), Health Education Kent Surrey Sussex Editorial Board Member, *Dental Nursing*

Career History 2006 Dental Nurse, Hamills Family Dental Practice, Kent

2008 Oral Health Promoter, NHS Medway

2010 Oral Health Improvement Practitioner, IDH, Kent

2010 Dental Nurse Advisor Infection Control, London

2011 Associate Lecturer/Guest Speaker (temporary), University of Kent

Professional Interests As a DCP member of the GDC Fitness to Practice Panel, I have become acutely aware of the need for effective educational activities that will support and promote high standards of dental professional practice and the delivery of high standards of patient care.

Since graduating in 2012, I have published a variety of articles aimed specifically at encouraging and promoting the development of dental nurses.

Selected Publications Nash, M. (2012). Reflective practice: a learning tool for dental nurses. *Dental Nursing*, 8(12), 804–807.

Nash, M. (2012). Mentoring: a learning relationship to foster change. *Dental Nursing*, 9(4), 216–221.

Nash, M. (2013). Developing influence to promote change. *Dental Nursing*, 9(7), 408–411.

Nash, M. (2013). Barriers to participation in CPD, education and development. *Dental Nursing*, 9(12), 717–721.

Career Highlight: MBE *Janine Brooks*

Mrs Jane Dalgarno

Profile Jane is a dental care professional committed to the advancement of dental nurse education. She has experience in developing and delivering both primary and post-registrant dental nursing qualifications. She represents dental nurses in the national arena, holding the position of seconded member for education to the British Association of Dental Nurses.

Education 1993 Certificate for Dental Surgery Assistants
1996 Certificate in Oral Health Education
1998 Certificate in Dental Sedation Nursing
2002 Further Education Teaching Certificates Stage 1 & 2
2004 A1/A2 City & Guilds Assessors Award
2008 Cert. Ed. Post Compulsory Education
2008 Certificate in Dental Radiography
2013 BSc Primary Dental Care (First Class Honours)
Current Roles Dental nurse tutor, CDS Community Interest Company social enterprise
Tempdent training and recruitment
National examiner for the Diploma, Oral Health and Sedation Certificates
DCP Affiliate member of FGDP(UK)
Member of Sedation Committee, National Examining Board for Dental Nurses
Member of the Local Dental Education Committee, Health Education East of England
Career History 1986 Dental nurse, general practice
1995 Senior dental nurse, community dental service
2007 Dental nurse tutor, Barnfield College
2012 HEE London Deanery
Professional Interests An active member of the British Association of Dental Nurses
Full member, Institute for Learning

Mrs Claudia Anne Peace

Profile Claudia is a general dental practitioner. Over the years, she has worked in the Royal Army Dental Corps and as an associate in five multihanded NHS practices across England and Northern Ireland. Her interests include providing composite restorations and root canal therapy.
Education 1981 BDS, Liverpool
Current Roles Associate General Dental Practitioner
Honorary Treasurer, Hants and Isle of Wight LDC
Dental Appraiser, Health Education Wessex
Career History 1982 Short Service Commission in Royal Army Dental Corps
1985 Associate, Multihanded NHS practice
1987 Associate, Multihanded NHS practice, Northern Ireland
Professional Interests Dental leadership and dental politics and a keen passion for clinical dentistry

Dr Manish Chitnis

Profile Manish is a general dental practitioner who has developed diverse interests. He has a strong network of dental colleagues and support staff and is passionate about his goals. In particular, he has a strong belief in striving for excellence in work and that success follows excellence. He has successfully run his own dental business in both the United Kingdom and India and enjoys delivering a mix of NHS, private and specialist dental care.

Education 1996 BDS Pune, India

2004 MFGDP, FGDP (UK)

2005 IQE, Eastman

2006 MFDS, Royal College of Surgeons and Physicians, Glasgow

2009 Business management in dentistry, BUOLD, Bristol

2011 Train the Trainers, Oxford

Current Roles General Dental Practitioner, Dental Corporate

Training Programme Director, HEE Thames Valley and Wessex

NHS England, Educational Assessments

Business Owner – Dental Concepts, mixed dental practice

Career History 1996 General Dental Practitioner, India

1997 Locum Associate Dentist, Mulund, India

1998 Practice Principal, Lead Dentist, Business Owner, India

2000 Opened Smile Specialty Clinic, India

2006 IQE Facilitator, ADP

2007 Area Clinical Manager, ADP

2011 Clinical Support Manager, IDH

Professional Interests Networking, quality assurance, standards, education. Dedication, determination and drive for achievement are his guides. His future next steps are into senior management and business partnership.

Mrs Jane Davies-Slowik

Profile Jane is a specialist in special care dentistry, associate postgraduate dental dean in the West Midlands and examiner for the Royal College of Surgeons. She is involved in dental politics.

Education 1980 BDS Liverpool

1988 Master of Community Dental Health

2010 Postgraduate Certificate in Education (distinction)

2014 ILM Level 7 Cert. in Executive Coaching and Mentoring

Current Roles Clinical Tutor, West Midlands Salaried Primary Care Dental Services

Associate Dental Dean, Dental Education (CPD) and Performance Development, HE West Midlands

Specialist Special Care Dentistry, Wolverhampton

Health Associate

Examiner for Diploma Special Care Dentistry, Royal College of Surgeons, England

Honorary Lecturer, Dental Public Health, University of Birmingham

Vice Chair, Local Dental Committee, Wolverhampton

Career History 1981 Community Dental Officer, Liverpool

1983 Salaried General Dental Practitioner, Liverpool

1984 Community Dental Officer, Dudley

1987 Senior Community Dental Officer, Dudley

1989 Assistant District Dental Officer, Dudley

1990 Acting District Dental Officer, Dudley

1993 Community Dental Services Manager, Dudley

1993 Secretary, West Midlands Division of CDS Group, BDA

1994 Chair of Midlands Society for the Study of Children's Dentistry

1995–96 Career Break

1996 Volunteer Dentist for Action health in Dharamsala, India

1996 General Manager, Professional Clinical Services, Dudley

1996 Clinical Director, Community Dental Services, Dudley

1996 Chair of the Liaison Group for Community Dental Practitioners

1997 Chair of the West Midlands Division of the CDS Group of the BDA

1998 First Elected Chair of Section of Clinical Community Dentistry, British Association Special Care Dentistry (BASCD)

1999 Clinical Director, Community Dental Services, Wolverhampton (0.5 wte)

2002 Retaining and Returning Adviser, West Midlands Deanery (0.2 wte)

2004 Chair of Wolverhampton Dental Advisory Group

2002/03 President Elect of British Association for the Study of Community Dentistry (BASCD)

2003/04 President of BASCD

> *Top Tip: Grasp every opportunity you can – you never know where it will lead you*
>
> Emma Worrell

Mr Steve Brookes

Profile Steve is a skilled GDP with postgraduate qualifications and interests in education, general dentistry and orthodontics. He works with the GDC Dental Complaints Service, Health Education Thames Valley and the LDC, and is clinical director lead for 44 practice locations. He has overall responsibility for day-to-day clinical governance, provides mentoring support and advice to over 300 dentists and handles complaints for Rodericks, a dental corporate.

Education 1984 BDS Guys Dental Hospital London
1985 LDS RCS Royal College of Surgeons of England
2001 MFGDP(UK) Faculty of General Dental Practitioners
2005 DPDS Bristol University Dental School
2009 Cert Med Ed Oxford Brookes University & NESC
Current Roles Clinical Director, Rodericks Ltd
Practice Principle
Training Programme Director, HEE Thames Valley Foundation Training
    Programme
GDC Expert Witness
GDC reports for Investigating Committee
Dental Complaints Service Professional Adviser
LDC Elected Member
Regional Vocational Training Committee Member
Dental Nurse Training Programme Tutor/Lecturer
Career History 1990 Vocational Trainer
1998 Orthodontic Clinical Assistant, Northampton
1998 Primary Care Trust Dental Discipline Committee Member
2000 Vocational Training Adviser, Oxford
2004 Dental Practice Adviser, Northampton
2008 Winner, Vocational Trainer of the Year
2009 Vocational Training Adviser, Northampton
Professional Interests Education

Mrs Geraldine Birks

Profile Geraldine is a dental nurse with a passion for education and quality.
    She also has a thirst for knowledge, most recently having completed her BA
    (Hons) in Education and Professional Development. She performs several
    roles for the GDC, is a deanery tutor, examiner for NEBDN and still finds
    time to be an independent trainer and lecturer.
Education 2002 NEBDN National Certificate in Dental Nursing
2003 NEBDN Dental Conscious Sedation
2004 City & Guilds 730-7 Adult Teaching Certificate
2005 NEBDN Certificate in Oral Health Education
2006 A1 Assessors Award
2007 City & Guilds Dental Nurse Licentiate (LCGI)
2008 & 2011 CIEH – Health & Safety Level 2
2009 CIEH – COSHH Level 2
2010 Diploma in Teaching in Lifelong Learning Sector – Full Diploma
BA (Hons) in Education & Professional Development, University of
    Huddersfield
Post Compulsory Certificate in Education, University of Huddersfield

Current Roles 2006 DCP Postgraduate Tutor, HEE Yorkshire & The Humber, Higher Education England, University of Leeds

2009 Fitness to Practice Investigating Committee Panel Member, GDC

2012 Quality Assurance Educational Inspector of UK Dental Schools, GDC

2006 Independent Lecturer/Trainer

2007 Examiner of the National Certificate in Dental Nursing and the Certificate in Oral Health Education. National Examining Board for Dental Nurses (NEBDN)

2013 Presiding Examiner of the NEBDN Certificate in Oral Health – Leeds

2014 Specialist Advisor, Care Quality Commission

2014 Registration Panel Assessor, GDC

Career History 2002 Dental Nurse Specialist, Hull PCT Salaried Dental Service

2006 Dental Nurse Tutor, York College

2008 NEBDN Quality Assurance Committee member

2011 Lead Dental Nurse Tutor, York College

Professional Interests Ethics, professionalism, quality, education, governance

Professor Sara Holmes MBE

Profile Sara is a truly inspirational individual. Her dental career began in dental nursing. Within 10 years, she had developed her skills and started down the path of educational studies. Over the years, she has built, managed and developed a number of successful learning and teaching innovation teams. She is currently director of the Portsmouth Dental Academy and received a personal chair (dental education) in 2014.

Education 1987 Dental Nursing, NEBDN

1995 Diploma, Oral Health Science and Education, University of Nottingham

1996 Certificate Adult Learning, University of Southampton

1996 Oral Health Education, NEBDN

1997 Post graduate Certificate, Education, Highbury College

1999 Diploma Conscious Sedation Nursing, NEBDN

2000 BSc Health Promotion (1st class), University of Portsmouth

2002 MSc Health Professional Education, University of Portsmouth

2012 Doctor of Education, University of Brighton

Current Roles Director, University of Portsmouth Dental Academy

Adjunct Professor, University of North Carolina

Personal Chair, Dental Education, University of Portsmouth

Editorial Board, *Primary Dental Journal*

Editorial Board, *Private Dentistry*

Editorial Board, *EC Dental Science*

Career History 1886 Dental Nurse, General Dental Practice

1991 Maxillofacial Nurse, Southampton City Hospital

1992 Dental Nurse, Emergency Dental Service

1996 Programme Director, Highbury College of Further & Higher Education

1997 Epidemiological Project Officer, Portsmouth Hospital Trust

1998 Lecturer/Senior Lecturer, Portsmouth Institute of Medicine & Healthcare, University of Portsmouth

2000 Secondment, Teaching Fellowship Lead, Dept. of Curriculum & Quality Enhancement, University of Portsmouth

2002 Director of Education, Portsmouth Institute of Medicine & Healthcare, University of Portsmouth

2004 Head of School, School of Professionals Complimentary to Dentistry, University of Portsmouth

2006 MBE

2008 External Examiner, University of Kent

2010 Direct of the University of Portsmouth Dental Academy

2010 Honorary Senior Lecturer King's College London

2010 GDC Expert Working Group (DCP Chair) – setting new standards for the QA of dental education in England, Northern Ireland, Scotland and Wales

2012 National Teaching Fellowship, Higher Education Academy

2014 Principal fellowship, Higher Education Academy

Professional Interests The relationship between health care policy and practice, training and education of the dental team, the future health care workforce

Mr Keith Ralph Percival

Profile Keith has a very active role in the largest LDC in the United Kingdom (Hampshire and Isle of Wight). He has also undertaken a number of roles in education and quality assurance, including selection panels for vocational trainers, regional advisors and postgraduate tutors.

Education 1971 BDS Birmingham

1988 MGDS RCS Eng

1993–95 – Orthodontic Module BUOLD Bristol

1994–95 – Clinical Audit Facilitator Training

2010 FFGDP (UK)

2011–12 – Coach/Mentor Training and Certification, Health Education Thames Valley and Wessex

Current Roles Chairman of the British Dental Guild

Committee Member British Society General Dental Surgery

Honorary LDC Secretary

Member of BDA Wessex Branch

Appraiser

Coach/Mentor supporting remediation programmes
Foundation Training by Equivalence Assessor
Elected General Dental Practice Committee (GDPC) Member for Hampshire
Honorary Treasurer BDA Golf Society
Career History 1972 General Dental Practitioner
1974 Partner with a Special Interest in Orthodontics
1993 Part-Time Clinical Assistant in Orthodontics
1995 Facilitator, Clinical Audit and Peer Review
1998 Honorary Secretary LDCs – Current LDC from 2007
2000 Elected GDSC Member for Hants and IoW LDC
2003 Elected GDPC Member for Hants and IoW LDC
2009 President Wessex BDA Branch Council
2011 Honorary LDC Secretary
2011 Honorary LDC Treasurer
Professional Interests Dental politics, education, remediation, governance

Mrs Nichola Peasnell

Profile Nicky is a senior lecturer at the University of Northampton. She is Year 1 lead for the Foundation Degree for Dental Nursing, the first of its kind in the United Kingdom. She lectures on the programme and is also admissions tutor. She began her career in dentistry as a dental nurse in general practice.
Education National Certificate in Dental Nursing – National Examination Board for Dental Nurses
Level 6 BSc in Profession Practice, Module: Facilitate Learning in Professional Practice
Level 6 BSc in Professional Practice Module: Transcultural Care
Level 6 BSc in Professional Practice Module: Reflective Practice
Level 6 BSc in Professional Practice Module: Research Methods
Fluoride Application – University of Portsmouth
Radiography – Northamptonshire Healthcare NHS Trust/West Midlands School of Radiography
Certificate in Oral Health Education, British Dental Association
Certificate in Impression Taking and Casting
Certificate in Suture Removal
NVQ Level 3 Customer Service – University of Northampton/Northampton Healthcare NHS Trust
Level 3 Assessors Award (D32/33) City & Guilds
Level 3 Work Place Coaching Institute of Leadership and Management
Level 4 Certificate in Further Education Teaching Stage 1
Level 4 Certificate in Further Education Teaching Stage 2
Level 4 Licentiateship Award Dental Nursing City & Guilds

Level 4 Certificate in Conducting Internal Quality Assurance (V1)
Level 4 Certificate in Leadership and Management – Work Place Coaching
BSc in Professional Practice, University of Northampton
Current Roles Senior Lecturer, University of Northampton
Dental Nurse, General Practice
Mentor
Career History 1980 Trainee Dental Nurse
1982 Dental Nurse
1988 Dental Practice Manager
1995 Dental Nurse
1997 Head Dental Nurse
2001 Assessor, Internal Verifier, Tutor
2007 Senior Lecturer
Professional Interests Education, quality assurance, mentoring and coaching, oral health education, continuing professional development

> **Top Tip:** *Get plenty of fresh air, look at the horizon, gather your thoughts*
> Janet Clarke

Dr May Hendry

Profile May is a general dental practitioner with broad experience in both clinical dentistry and dental leadership. Currently, her two main roles are as a principal in general dental practice and as dental practice adviser (DPA).
Education 1982 BDS (with commendation) Glasgow
1998 MFGDP(UK)
Current Roles Practice Owner and GDP
Dental Practice Adviser, NHS Ayrshire and Arran.
Member of the Quality Improvement in Dentistry Group (appointment by invitation from the Scottish Government)
Chair of Quality Improvement and Supporting Practice Group (appointment by invitation from the Scottish Government).
Career History 1982 House Officer, Glasgow Dental Hospital
1983 (to present) Associate Positions in General Dental Practice
1984 Clinical Assistant, Department of Conservative Dentistry, Glasgow Dental Hospital and School
1990 Visiting Dental Surgeon, Marks and Spencer, Ayr
1991 Honorary Clinical Lecturer, University of Glasgow, Department of Conservative Dentistry
1993 Practice owner and practising GDP, Troon, Ayrshire
1994 Member of the Scottish Dental Practice Board (5-year appointment by invitation from the Scottish Office)

1996 Clinical assessor for NHS Scotland Complaints Procedure (appointment by invitation from the Scottish Office)

1998 Member of Readers' Panel for Dental Update

2000 Member of the Scottish Dental Vocational Training Appeals Body (appointment by invitation from the Scottish Executive)

2000 President of the Ayrshire Dental Society (1-year appointment by invitation from the society)

2001 Chairman of the Primary Care Dental Practice Accreditation Group: Clinical Standards Board for Scotland (appointment by invitation from the Clinical Standards Board for Scotland)

2004 Joint Chairman of the NHS Quality Improvement Scotland and National Care Standards Committee Dental Services Standards Working Group (appointment by invitation from NHS Quality Improvement Scotland)

2007 Chairman of the Scottish Dental Practice Advisers Group

2008 Member of the Review of Statement of Dental Remuneration Group (appointment by invitation from the Scottish Government)

2011 Member of the Working Group for the West of Scotland Managed Network in Restorative Dentistry

Professional Interests Special clinical interest in advanced restorative dentistry

Within the DPA role, an interest in quality improvement in dentistry

Conclusion

Those I have included in this chapter are a very small sample of the amazing people who work in dentistry across a wide and diverse portfolio of roles and responsibilities. They are talented individuals, and each and every one of them inspires me. I hope their stories and CVs have conveyed the immense variety of opportunities that we as dental professionals have available to us. I thank them all for their generosity in helping their colleagues.

> *You miss 100% of the shots you don't take*
>
> Wayne Gretzky

Chapter 6 Networking and networks

```
C H A N G E       G L U E
V     E           I
      T W O       I N V E S T
      W     V     K         I
      C O N T A C T S       M
      R     L         T     E
W O R K     S U P P O R T
A     S     E         U
Y O U       G I V E
```

Top Tip: *Learn to listen, as good ideas can come from the most unlikely sources*

Derek Richards

In this chapter, I will be covering networks and the importance of networking in developing and progressing your career. There will be some tips on how to network successfully and how to construct a network map. In addition, I have included a section on writing a curriculum vitae and how to tailor it to the job you are applying for.

> *All you need are curiosity and a willingness to meet others. I believe that every single person I come across has something interesting to say.*
>
> Julia Hobsbawn

City University London, Cass Business School appointed Julia Hobsbawn as visiting professor in networking in December 2011 – how great is that? Personally, I think the recognition that networking is a skill – a valuable skill and one we can all develop and benefit from – is such a validation.

Julia goes on to say:

> *During 30 years I have built up my own networks to draw on, stretching from London to New York, from politics to academia. How did I get to be the world's first professor in networking? Yes, of course: my networks.*

How to Develop Your Career in Dentistry, First Edition. Janine Brooks.
© 2015 John Wiley & Sons, Ltd. Published 2015 by John Wiley & Sons, Ltd.

Networks are essential. They can save your sanity, help your career move forward and keep you on the right track. Networking was another lesson I learnt very early on in my career, again from Bob Izon when I worked in Hereford. The county had an excellent dental society at that time – and probably still does. It had regular meetings, which most of the Herefordshire dentists attended. I met and got to know my colleagues soon after I started work and this helped me enormously when making patient referrals or discussing service developments. Just being able to pick up the telephone to ask advice from a colleague was a great support, especially in my first few years. Getting to know people outside work made working with them so much easier. We even had a county-wide out-of-hours service in which everyone took part, salaried and general practice – virtually unheard of in those days.

However, local networks were not enough, and Bob suggested that if I really wanted to get on in my career I needed to attend the BDA meetings and the CDS group meetings. This meant travelling to Birmingham, a 100-mile round trip for the evening. Driving up to Birmingham after a long surgery session along winding country lanes was unappealing to say the least, particularly in the winter, but I kept going. Of course, Bob was right: the people I met then are still friends and colleagues now, over 30 years on. A lesson about networks: they are like the theme tune for Neighbours: 'Good network colleagues can become good friends.' If this sounds a bit corny, it might be, but networks and networking work. Through my networks, I found out about opportunities for work, I learnt from colleagues' experiences and I received good advice when dealing with problems or difficult issues. A good network, carefully nurtured, gives a safe, nonjudgemental place in which to share your strengths and weaknesses with trusted colleagues, get feedback and support and realise that most of the problems you come across have already been experienced and solved by someone else. My closest network began in the 1990s, when I took the Masters in Community Dental Health (MCDH) at Birmingham Dental School. There were seven of us – I'd like to say we resembled the Magnificent Seven, but that would be stretching the truth rather considerably. We did become a very cohesive group, and to this day four of us meet regularly both inside and outside work. I consider them to be my closest colleagues, friends and confidants.

You could begin to broaden your network by collecting the contact details of interesting people you meet: who they are, where they work, what experience they have and where you met them. Why? Dentistry, and even general health care, is a small place: we seem particularly good at recycling people. You will meet the same people again and again; these will be the people who help you as you progress through your career, and who you contact for advice. You never know when something new will present itself and you will want to talk to someone experienced in a particular field. They might introduce you to others who can give you advice, guidance or even a job. If nothing else, your network will sustain you when the going gets tough – and from time to time, the going will get tough. Because of the way dentistry mostly operates – through the direct care and treatment of patients – it can be a little lonely; even isolated. For that reason, dental professionals need to make a conscious effort to network and spend time with colleagues. It's good for you, good for your patients and good for the profession – what's not to like?

People you network with can act as informal mentors – sometimes even coaches. You will be surprised what you can learn from even the shortest conversation.

> **Top Tip:** *Be positive – the glass is half full*
>
> Bal Chana

How do you network?

You've already started. If you are at the beginning of your career (lucky you) then you have your network of fellow students, foundation trainees and work colleagues. If you are part way through your career (lucky you) then you have your work colleagues – not only current, but from previous jobs – and perhaps BDA members, BADN members or other specialist societies. Networking takes effort (very little of value doesn't): you need to begin conversations, maintain contacts and be prepared to give as much as you hope to get back. Networks don't have to be just about work – they will usually begin that way, but the best and most sustained networks have an element of the social to them. Inevitably, when dental professionals get together, even socially, we talk about dentistry, so the opportunity to support each other is always there. You can find a number of good books (and some not so good) on networking, and I do not intend to go into minute detail here. I have listed some that you may find useful at the end of this chapter. However, I will outline some of the basics of networking here, as I feel it is a core skill for your career. These are my top ten tips for growing and sustaining a great network.

1. Be prepared to work at it
Networking and keeping up with your networks takes time and effort, and if you are not prepared to put either in then you are unlikely to reap the rich rewards from networks. Networks require give and take and investment, particularly at the beginning. Very little that is worthwhile does not need work.

2. Don't be afraid to take the initiative
Networks are two-way: the people you network with will value you just as much as you value them. We all have things to offer each other. So, don't be

afraid to go up to someone, introduce yourself and ask them about themselves or about the conference or meeting you are both attending. Start the ball rolling. Be curious about other people: it's not just about you. The more you listen, the more you learn.

3. Give as much (at least) as you get

Help people that you network with – give them links to information you have and people you know. Networks take time to grow and mature; the help you give today may translate into a brilliant introduction for a job in the future. Good networks do not happen overnight.

4. Know that you are networking

Some people are naturals at building a network of friends and colleagues with seemingly little effort. However, most of us need to work at it, certainly in the beginning. Be positive and purposeful about building your network. Go to meetings, go to conferences and talk to people, seek them out. Talk to people you have already met and refresh the network, and talk to people you haven't met and grow the network. When you are growing your virtual network online, know who you want to link with; for example, professionals in your specialty, your geographic location or your area of dentistry. Have a collecting policy and be discriminating.

5. Know why you are networking

Networks help us to become better known and better connected and increase our knowledge. They are a good thing, but to get the most from them you need to know you are networking and not just have a social chit chat. Decide what you want to know and what you want to achieve, and specifically introduce yourself to people who might be able to help you. But – and here is a real secret of networking – be spontaneous, because sometimes meeting new people is fortuitous: you don't know who they are until you start talking to them, and then you find they are a mine of information and they have great contacts – and hopefully you like them, as well. Such people are the real pearls of networking. At its core, networking is about making connections with others that might benefit you both. Have a plan, but don't be afraid to deviate from it if a new opportunity comes along.

6. Invest in networking

Networking is like any development: it takes investment. Networking is building for the future, and it requires you to spend time and money now for reward in the future. Your investment will be worth it – maybe not today, maybe not tomorrow, but it will be worth it. Do not expect your networking to be confined to work hours. Invest time in yourself outside routine hours:

go to evening meetings, be prepared to use the odd weekend to network – it will be worth it. Do not expect a network to come to you: you have to go out and make it.

7. Use different methods

The method you use will depend on the type of network you are seeking. Face-to-face and electronic networking are both good. Meetings, conferences and the practice are good places to network. So is LinkedIn. Personally, I like to start by networking face to face. I find you gain so much more information from interacting with people in the same room – listening to their voices, watching their expressions and body language. Once contact has been made, electronic methods can kick in, and these can be very successful in maintaining networks.

8. Keep notes

If you are keen to build your network, you need to keep notes. I don't mean making notes while you are talking to people. I don't mean making it some sort of academic endeavour. I mean keeping a record of who you meet and where and writing down their contact details – email addresses and telephone numbers are the most useful. Then you can contact them in the future if there is a new career opportunity you are interested in. If you want to be scientific, you could draw a network map (see later). These are excellent aide memoirs, showing who you know and where they are in your network. Often, people will belong to a number of organisations – you might have worked with them before.

9. Relationship building

The best networks are built on mutual respect and social glue. This is about the future, and you will find that it really is who you know and what they know about you that matters. The people in your network will have networks of their own. People you know will remember you and talk about you to other people, perhaps recommending they contact you about interesting projects or opportunities.

10. Be true: build your reputation

Develop your profile and invest in your self-development. Be a person worth networking with. You need to be more than a self-publicist: you need to have substance. If someone trusts you then their contacts will be influenced by the way they talk about you. As I have said before, networking is about give and take; it's about what you can contribute as much as what you can get back.

> **Top Tip:** *Most people are worth knowing*
>
> Janine Brooks

What networking should not be

- selling;
- making a pitch;
- exploitation;
- a chore; or
- trading business cards.

Networking, at its heart, should be an enjoyable activity: it is positive. You are not trying to find out information so that you can undercut someone in a business deal. Its primary aim should not be to sell. A benefit of networks is that business opportunities often arise. Once people know about you, what you do and what you can offer, they are much more likely to want to work with you and tell other people about you. However, if you enter a networking relationship with the sole aim of sell, sell, sell you will not be authentic and your network may be short-lived. No one likes to be exploited, and successful networks do not exploit individuals. If you really find introducing yourself to new people or asking people about themselves and being genuinely interested in them difficult and a chore then networking, and certainly face-to-face networking, is unlikely to be for you. It's natural to be a bit nervous at first, and this is where a mentor can be very helpful: they can introduce you to a network and smooth the ground initially. Finally, networking is not about a cold exchange of business cards. Of course, exchanging contact details is part of networking, but it's not speed dating for dental professionals. Make sure you do have cards with your contact details on them to give to people, but don't thrust them in their face or pocket and think that you have networked – at best you have just been a bit irritating, at worst people will avoid you in future.

> **Career Highlight:** *FFGDP(UK) by election*
>
> Janine Brooks

Where can you network?

There is no one place: it's wherever you meet people. You network at work, at professional meetings, at conferences, on committees, online. LinkedIn is a professional network and is good for looking up people who have experiences you would like to know more about. Join professional or specialist societies, go to their meetings and talk to people. People love to be asked about what they do. People generally like to be asked for their advice or opinion. Most people like to help fellow professionals.

After you have met someone who you get on with particularly well or who has shared some piece of interesting information, you might email them or contact them through LinkedIn. This keeps you on their network radar.

> **Top Tip:** *Always have a purpose in life*
>
> Bal Chana

Types of network

We are all networkers; we just choose whether to be good at it or not so good. Choose to make networking work for you.

Knowing who to go to for advice and to get information from is one of the most important skills you can develop. Making contacts widely gives you a head start when taking your career in a new direction. The table below discribes different types of network.

Table 6.1 Types of network

Type	Function/characteristics
Support	A nonjudgmental network in which you can give and receive constructive, honest feedback. The network often challenges you, but in a good, stretching way. Such networks often consist of close colleagues, family and friends.
Current job	This network consists of the people who can help you be the best you can be. They might be senior, experienced colleagues who can mentor you and help you build your reputation. These are the people who will give you experience and the projects that build your skills for the present and the future.
Future career opportunities	This is a network of 'gatekeepers': people who know about job opportunities or who are doing the sort of job you are interested in. They can help you make up your mind about whether a job is really what you think it is. They may be able to open doors to where the jobs are and introduce you to other influential people you can talk to.
Linking	This is a network of people with information and who are well connected themselves. They can introduce you to other useful people.

Electronic networks

So far, I've mostly written about physical networking. Electronic networks are also useful. I imagine most people reading this will have at least some electronic networks: Facebook, Twitter, LinkedIn and so on. There will be some who have not used these technologies yet, but surprisingly few.

There are over 250 social and professional networking Web sites and fora that you can join. The majority are social sites, such as Facebook, Faceparty and Google+. However, there are specific professional and business networks that can be of help in building your contacts and networks and you might want to think about them. If used well, they can complement your physical networking. Table 6.2 lists a few sites you might consider joining.

Personally, I use LinkedIn as a 'shop window' to let contacts know what I have done, what I'm currently doing and important pieces of work I have completed. I have gained work through LinkedIn and I have used it to find speakers for conferences and training I have organised. There are specific interest groups you can join within LinkedIn, such as specific professional groups, leadership groups and dental business groups. You can easily set up your own group, too, whether open or closed.

Twitter is not a network in the same sense as those in Table 6.2, but it can be a useful way of sending messages to people who follow you and it does have a useful business and professional function. I have a Twitter account and I

Table 6.2 Networking Web sites

Web site	Purpose
Academia.eu	Academic sharing/research
Bebo	General
Epernicus	Research scientists
Facebook	General
Faceparty	General
Focus.com	Business-to-business, worldwide
Google+	General
LinkedIn	Business and professional networking
MySpace	General
Talkbiznow	General business networking
Yammer	Social networking for work colleagues
WebDental	Professional networking for dental professionals
GDPUK	Professional networking and information site for dental professionals
NewDocs	Professional networking for dental professionals
Dentalcompanies	Professional networking

do tweet for business/professional use, although not as much as I might do. It can be useful for sending links, short messages and information on your LinkedIn account or another Web site you have.

> **Top Tip:** *Do to others as you would like done unto yourself*
>
> Shazad Malik

Network map

Drawing a network map can help you visualise where your networks are and how they relate to one another. They can be very useful when you are trying to think who to contact and where to go for advice. To help you when constructing your own map, I have provided an example in Figure 6.1. You can choose to draw your map in any form you want: you could use concentric circles, with you as the centre circle; you could give each person, job, organisation a separate box; you could group categories differently. What is important is that you try to include as much as possible from your past and present: this is the solid foundation for the future.

My map looks crowded, and so it should after a working career of over 40 years (I've included both my pre-dental and my post-dental life). It would look a lot more crowded if I had included individuals or tried to show the links between the categories and within the categories. My map is a 'core' map: it shows on one page all the contacts and networks I have developed and that I could use if I were looking for new information. Let me give you an illustration of how a network works: I started as a postgraduate at Birmingham University, where I met six other people. In the intervening years we saw each other at meetings and conferences, and four of us meet socially. In 2002 I was looking for something different, and one of these people told me about an opportunity they had heard of with a national organisation. I hadn't known about it – I must have missed the advertisement. I applied for the job and got it.

Another example comes from someone I worked with. She had been asked to be part of an interview panel, but the panel didn't appoint. She told the chief executive that she knew someone who would be right for the job. They contacted me, we met up, I applied for the job and I got it. Networks work.

Networking facilitates you in making and nurturing meaningful relationships. Those relationships will have a number of functions: career development, career support, personal support, collaboration. They can include all of these and more.

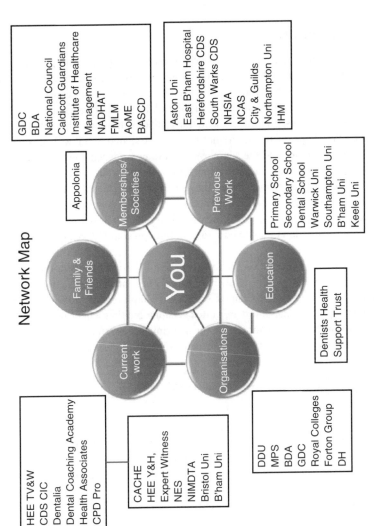

Figure 6.1 Network map.

As your network grows and your contacts begin to work for you in career development, it is essential that you have an up-to-date CV. I have included a short section on CVs next to help you when you are thinking of giving yours a refresh.

Curriculum vitae

A curriculum vitae is essential for your career development and planning. You need to begin building your CV from the moment you start to think about looking for jobs. From then on, keep it up to date. Have a core CV that includes everything you have done. Include all the jobs you have undertaken: the responsibilities, projects, presentations and qualifications. This will grow to be a very large document. It's not meant to be shared in full with anyone; it is your reference and the source you will draw on when you tailor a CV for a specific job. Every job you apply for throughout your career must have a tailored CV, which must match the essential requirements of the job and as many of the desirable requirements as possible. The people responsible for screening CVs ahead of shortlisting want their job to be as straightforward as possible – they don't want to have to hunt through your CV to find shortlisting criteria.

You can find information on how to write a CV, what format to use, how long it should be from a number of places. There are many examples and templates you can look at. Chapter 5 contains examples of CVs from a number of dental professionals; most are potted versions, but they will help you when you are either writing your CV for the first time or refreshing it as you move though your career. I have also provided a short example CV in Figure 6.2.

> **Top Tip:** *Sleep and eat well; get into a good routine*
>
> Emma Worrell

This format is useful to showcase where you have been and a little of what you have done, but it does not demonstrate much about you or your capabilities. Another format, known as a functional DV, does do that: it takes its format from the person specification of the post you are applying for. It uses the headings of the person specification as hooks on which to hang information about how you demonstrate a particular skill or experience. Use the first person when writing a functional CV. An example is given in Figure 6.3: the person specification criteria are given in bold at the beginning of each section, then how they are met. I have purposely chosen a nonclinical post, because it can be harder to think how you meet the criteria in such cases. The functional CV is formatted in a way that says what you have done, not just who

Amelia Jones

Profile

A profile is a short showcase: a potted glimpse of you. Keep it punchy and use strong, action words to get the attention of the person shortlisting. Try to keep to under 100 words.

A senior clinical leader with 15 years' broad clinical and leadership experience in the National Health Service. Proven track record of effective leadership and motivation of staff. Ability to problem solve and tack around issues to achieve results. A first-class communicator accustomed to high-profile work and public speaking. Relishes new situations and fresh opportunities. Excellent network links both within and external to the NHS.

Current Roles
Put in all your current paid and honorary positions. Include the month and year you took up the post.

Blankshire
Associate   Aug 2011 to date

General Dental Council
Quality Assurance Education Inspector   April 2006 to date

Dentists Health Support Trust
Trustee (Honorary)   Jan 2013 to date

Previous Roles (Last 10 Years)
I recommend only including jobs/roles you have undertaken in the last 10 years to maintain currency. Longer than that and you are probably out of date. This should not be a list of all your jobs since leaving school or training. Begin with the most recent role and work backwards. That way, your latest experience is noted first.

Blankshire
Institute of Health Care Management
Facilitator/Assessor – Accredited Manager Programme   April 2011 – Jan 2014

University of Dundee
Visiting Fellow in Dental Education   Aug 2000 – Aug 2011

City & Guilds
External Verifier (oral healthcare) (10 days per year)   Feb 2003 to Dec 2007

Dental Vocational Training Authority
Equivalence Committee Member (4 days per year)   May 2001 to Mar 2005

Figure 6.2 Sample curriculum vitae.

Educational History

Include your pre-registrant training and any postgraduate or post-registration training. Do not include continuing professional development. You do not need to include pre-University (school) qualifications.

1. Undergraduate

B.D.S. University of Birmingham   1996–2000

2. Postgraduate

Diploma in Dental Public Health Royal College of Surgeons,   2005
London

Postgraduate Certificate in Medical Education, University of   2007
Warwick

Honours

Fellowship by election to the Faculty of General Dental Practice   2010
(UK), Royal College of Surgeons (London)

Publications

You should be selective here. Include publications relevant to the job you are applying for or those in the last 10 years.

Academic Papers

Pacer, E.R., Prancer, D.A. and Dancer, J. (2008). A review of present delivery in the UK. *Community Dental Health*, **20**, 16, PNID 12688599.

White, R., Black, K.A. and Green, J. (2011). An investigation into the numbers of dentists from 19 European Economic Area (EEA) receiving socks for Christmas. *British Dental Journal*, **11**(3), 13–17.

Book

Jones, A. (2010). *Toothbrushes: The Ideal Gift for the Man who has Everything.* Lambert Academic Publishing.

Memberships

Academy of Medical Educators – Fellow
Royal College of Surgeons of London
Faculty of General Dental Practice
British Association of Community Dentistry

Significant Projects

In this section, choose projects and pieces of work you have completed that are relevant to the job you are applying for. They should be pieces of work you have personally undertaken or those you have led. Say what you did, how you did it and what the result was. Do not include a job description: it says nothing about what you actually do.

Figure 6.2 (*continued*)

Post applied for: CQC member

Senior level expertise, ideally of working in the commercial sector in a service industry with a significant level of achievement in his or her chosen field

As Associate Director of Dentistry I am strategic lead for dentistry, responsible for developing and implementing the dental programme across England, Scotland, Wales and Northern Ireland. I advise the senior management team on all aspects of dentistry and contribute to the effective strategic development and management of the organisation.

I oversaw the integration of the adviser team, whereby all advisers regardless of their professional background were enabled to work with any referral. We now offer a full advice, support and assessment service for all NHS dentists. This has involved considerable leadership skills and the ability to push forward change and new ideas. The model I developed was used as the template for our expansion to work with opticians.

Commercially and politically aware with the ability to understand and translate the impact of external factors in the context of CQC

Since graduation in December 2000 I have worked within the NHS. In that time there have been several reorganisations instigated by government policy. Over the years, as my roles have moved from local to regional to national, my knowledge of government has grown. I regularly meet with the section of the Department of Health that has most influence on my current area of work. Of all the health professional groups, I believe dentistry to be the most commercially aware, and while I have worked within the employed sector, my roles have required frequent contact and liaison with independent practitioners, most of whom operated within a commercial culture.

My work at the NHS Information Authority (NHSIA) allowed me to develop my commercial and political awareness. The NHSIA was formed from a number of organisations and retained a distinct commercial flavour.

Figure 6.3 Functional CV.

The ability to address high-profile, complex and sensitive issues in a way that represents individual and wider public feeling

The work I do with partnership organisations and key stakeholders is totally developmental and nonhierarchical. The organisation is not a regulator, and being able to facilitate partnership working is essential to our success.

As part of my role in South Blankshire, I led the successful merger of two rehabilitation hospitals, for one of which I was general manager. This was a complex project and included planning new buildings and accommodation on one site while closing the other (my site). Public and staff consultation was an important part of the process and was continuous over the period. The whole process from initial planning to final move took almost three years. It was my responsibility to manage the development and ensure it met all national and local requirements and was completed to strict guidelines that were externally applied.

Excellent interpersonal communication skills, with the ability to lead, influence, inspire and challenge

My role in providing direct expert professional advice and support required extensive active listening and reflective skills to elicit the exact nature of concerns. In addition, it was important to use questioning skills, as often the person who made initial contact had little knowledge of dentistry. This type of work requires considerable tact and diplomacy, as the issues are usually complex and sensitive.

Demonstrable experience of successfully improving and managing organisational performance in a board-level position

In July 2002, I was appointed as Caldicott Guardian for the NHS Information Authority (five sessions per week), having previously undertaken the role in South Blankshire since April 1999. I delegated responsibility for the organisation's correct handling of patient identifiable data, including disclosure. I was directly responsible to the Chief Executive and advised the Board on all aspects of processing patient identifiable data. I was responsible for ensuring that all products, services and projects developed and managed by the Information Authority complied with legal and ethical guidance to include the Caldicott guidelines. National databases included the NHS Strategic Tracing Service, NHS number programme, Nationwide

Figure 6.3 (*continued*)

Clearing Service and Open Exeter systems. On a day-to-day basis, I supported and advised NHSIA staff on individual cases of confidentiality and disclosure of information. It was my responsibility to authorise disclosure of confidential patient data; many of the complex disclosure cases required close liaison with the NHSIA solicitors and occasional court appearances.

Sound experience of strategic planning, risk management and high-performance management

My day-to-day work is immersed in regulation and governance – clinical, professional, informational, the legal aspects of performance, data, confidentiality, risk and performance.

My contribution to the wider aspects of my organisation includes taking a lead in professional governance and ensuring that each aspect of the services is linked and that lessons are learnt across the organisation. I am Programme Director for Information Governance and successfully led the implementation of the Cabinet Office modernisation agenda for information governance.

Communication and conduct during hearings

I understand the seven Nolan principles (the Standards for Public Life) and have endeavoured to adhere to them throughout my professional career. They are particularly pertinent to my roles with national organisations, including the NHS Information Authority, City & Guilds, NCAS and the GDC. At all times, I am aware of the need to conduct myself in a manner consistent with the principles of selflessness, integrity, objectivity, accountability, openness, honesty and leadership, both personally and professionally. I believe I have in the past and that I continue to do so; it is important to my credibility within national governance frameworks that my actions are judged against these principles.

Figure 6.3 (*continued*)

you worked for. This is much more helpful to the people who will be shortlisting applications and it improves your chances of being asked to an interview considerably.

I have a number of CVs. I have one – the core CV – that I put everything into. This contains all my experience over the years: the jobs I have done, significant projects I've worked on, articles I've written, presentations I've made. I keep it up to date regularly, and it is now very long. I never use this CV when I'm applying for a job or a new project. Its usefulness to me is that I don't forget work that I have completed – and believe me, that can happen as your career progresses. I use it to construct CVs tailored to what I need them for. This also means I can put together a relevant CV very quickly should I need to.

Twenty years from now you will be more disappointed by the things that you didn't do than by the ones you did do. So, throw off the bowlines, sail away from the safe harbor. Catch the trade winds in your sails. Explore. Dream. Discover.

H. Jackson Brown's mother

Chapter 7 **Training and qualifications**

```
      C  A  T  S
N        R        M              F  F  D
V     M  A        S        D           D
Q  U  A  L  I  F  I  C  A  T  I  O  N  S
      S  N        N        P
      T  I     P  H  D     L  L  M
O  H  E  N                 O
      R  G                 M  R  E  S
                        B  A
```

> **Top Tip:** *Learn to take, blend and create; sometimes the most unlikely job leads to great things*
>
> Janine Brooks

Education is not an affair of telling and being told, but an active and constructive process.

Dewey (1916)

In this chapter, you will find information about some of the training and post-registration qualifications available to you. I have also included a section on how to develop and build your experience. The training and qualifications given in this chapter are mostly post-registration. Some are specific to a registrant group, but many are available and relevant across the profession. Because dentistry is an escalator profession (professionals may qualify for one registrant group and then later qualify for another), I have included some basic information about initial qualifications, although I have kept this brief. The chapter will concentrate on specific programmes of training and not continuing professional development or day courses. However, some shorter courses are included, such as commissioning, fluoride varnish application and mentoring. I do not try to be comprehensive, merely to give you a flavour

---

How to Develop Your Career in Dentistry, First Edition. Janine Brooks.
© 2015 John Wiley & Sons, Ltd. Published 2015 by John Wiley & Sons, Ltd.

of the considerable variety and breadth of what is available to dental professionals who wish to enrich their careers. Finally, I have included a short section on how to broaden and develop your experience.

In 2013, the BDA undertook some interesting market research into postgraduate qualifications and found that approximately 40% of GDP members in England and Wales had one (Anon, 2014). Those respondents under the age of 35 years were a little more likely to indicate they had a postgraduate qualification (45.5%) than those over 35; respondents over the age of 65 years had the lowest proportion (35.3%). It is interesting that older respondents were less likely to hold a postgraduate qualification. This might just be a sign of the times and that today's dentistry strongly encourages professionals to continue to acquire formal learning. While this study of 1117 BDA members may not be academically robust, it does indicate useful themes and suggests that a relatively high proportion of the dental profession undertakes post-registration study. Of course, it may well be that BDA members are more likely to undertake post-registration study than non-BDA members or that those BDA members who had post-registration qualifications were more likely to respond to the survey.

Postgraduate qualifications are usually subdivided into categories:

* **Certificate:** for example, Cert Med Ed, PGCert.
* **Diploma:** for example, PGDip, DPDS.
* **Master:** for example, MCDH, MSc.
* **PhD/Professional Doctorate:** for example, DDS, DMedEth.

Certificates and diplomas are often constructed in units of study and can build into a masters degree or remain as standalone accredited units. A PhD is a doctor of philosophy and will generally entail writing a dissertation of between 80 000 and 100 000 words of original research. Often, students begin their studies as an MPhil and convert to a PhD after satisfactory progress. Professional doctorates are equivalent to a PhD, but their focus is on a specific professional context. PhDs and professional doctorates are the highest levels of degree attainable within the United Kingdom. They require study of 3 years full time or 6 years part time. A masters degree generally requires 3 years' part-time study; full-time degrees are available and can be completed in a shorter amount of time.

Credit accumulation transfer schemes

Credit accumulation transfer schemes (CATS) use points to allow students to transfer learning and qualifications obtained from one educational institution to another and to credit them against another qualification. One credit point is the equivalent of 10 hours' notional learning time. This scheme began in the early 1990s. Generally, you can apply to transfer credits for study you have completed in the last 16 years; anything older than that is not eligible for credit transfer. You often find that postgraduate study programmes are made up of modules that are either 30 or 60 credits. This allows you to build your qualification and is well suited to the busy professional who fits their postgraduate study around work and home commitments.

Clinical programmes

Apart from the actual programmes, there is a wide variety of format delivery, from full-time face-to-face to part-time distance learning. The variety means you are sure to find a format that suits your life style, learning style and time availability. In this chapter, you will find taster information: I have not included every programme in every discipline provided by every educational provider. Not all courses are offered each year and new courses are being added every year, with some programmes being either revised or removed. I will give you signposts so that you can look in more detail for the topic, programme or course you wish to pursue.

- **MJDF RCS Eng.:** Diploma of Membership of the Joint Dental Faculties at the Royal College of Surgeons of England. Joint Exam. Two written examinations and a portfolio of evidence. www.rcseng.ac.uk/fds/mjdf.
- **MSc, MClinDent:** Conservative Dentistry, Endodontics, Implant Dentistry, Oral Medicine, Prosthetic Dentistry and Special Care Dentistry, Oral Surgery, Clinical Dentistry, Experimental Oral Pathology, Advanced General Dental Practice.
- **PhD:** Biomaterials Science and Dental Technology, Endodontology, Fixed and Removal Prosthodontics.
- **MPhil:** Dental Public Health/Community Dentistry, Oral Radiology, Orthodontics.
- **MD(Res):** Health Service and Population Research, Dental and Oral Health Care Sciences (Clinical Dentistry), Age-Related Diseases.
- **Diplomas:** Advanced Certificate in Aesthetic Dentistry, Implant Dentistry, Restorative Dentistry, Primary Care Orthodontics, Primary Dental Care, Dental Clinical Sciences.
- **Certificates:** Appraisal of Dental Practices, Dental Health Services Leadership and Management, Management Studies, Dental Implantology, Restorative Cosmetic Dentistry, Periodontology, Restorative Dental Practice.

> **Top Tip:** *Life is a journey with many ups and downs*
>
> Shazad Malik

National Vocational Qualifications (Levels 2–5)

These courses are available in a variety of formats, some distance learning, some blended (online and face to face). Most can be undertaken part time. Some are on-the-job based, such as an internal verifiers award.

- Business and Administration.
- Oral Health Care.
- Customer Care.
- Assessor Awards (D32/D33).
- Training & Development.
- Award Institute of Leadership and Management – Work Place Coaching.
- Certificate in Leadership and Management – Work Place Coaching.
- Internal Verifiers Award (D34).
- Certificate in Conducting Internal Quality Assurance (V1).

Expanded duties training

Most of these are short courses – some only a few days' intensive study. They will include practical and theoretical elements. Often you will need to be working with patients to gain a portfolio of practical experience.

- Certificate in Oral Health Education.
- Application of Topical Fluoride.
- Impression Taking.
- Removal of Sutures and Wound Healing.
- Dental Radiography.
- Dental Conscious Sedation.
- Certificate in Dental Sedation Nursing.
- Dental Photography.

> *The important thing is not to stop questioning. Curiosity has its own reason for existing*
>
> Albert Einstein

Non-clinical programmes

> *Top Tip:* Forgive
>
> Sophie Noske

All dental schools (and many other universities and higher education establishments) provide post-registration training programmes for dental registrants. Tables 7.1 and 7.2 give you examples of the postgraduate courses on offer. It is not exhaustive or comprehensive. Contact details are given for each

Table 7.1 Providers of post-registration training

Dental school	Contact details	Examples of courses
Aberdeen University Office King's College Aberdeen AB24 3FX	Tel: 01224 273 504 Fax: 01224 272 034 email: sras@abdn.ac.uk www.abdn.ac.uk/sras	PgCert Research Methods for Health by Online Learning PgCert Medical Education
Belfast Queen's University Belfast University Road Belfast BT7 1NN	Tel: 02890 973 838 Fax: 02890 975 151 email: admissions@qub.ac.uk www.qub.ac.uk	Master Public Health PGCert/PGDip/MSc Clinical Education
Birmingham The University of Birmingham Edgbaston Birmingham B15 2TT	Tel: 0121 415 8900 Fax: 0121 414 7159 email: admissions@bham.ac.uk www.bham.ac.uk	MSc in Advanced General Dental Practice
Bristol University of Bristol Undergraduate Admissions Office Senate House Tyndall Avenue Bristol BS8 1TH	Tel: 0117 928 9000 Fax: 0117 925 1424 email: ug-admissions@bristol .ac.uk www.bristol.ac.uk	MSc Dental Implantology MSc or Diploma Postgraduate Dental Studies DDS Orthodontics Research MSc and PhD BUOLD – Dental Postgraduate Studies – PGCert/ PGDip/MSc: Anxiety Management Business Management Skills Law and Ethics Local Anaesthesia Endodontics Periodontics Surgical Skills 1
Cardiff Cardiff University Newport Road Cardiff CF24 0DE	Tel: 02920 879 999 Fax: 02920 876 138 email: admissions@cardiff.ac.uk www.cardiff.ac.uk	PgCert/PgDip/MSc Medical Education MClinDent Clinical Dentistry MSc/PgDip: Conscious Sedation in Dentistry Implantology Tissue Engineering MScD Orthodontics Research degrees (PhD/MPhil/MScD): Tissue Engineering and Reparative Dentistry Applied Clinical Research and Public Health

(continued overleaf)

Table 7.1 (*continued*)

Dental school	Contact details	Examples of courses
Dundee University of Dundee Dundee DD1 4HN	Tel: 01382 383 838 Fax: 01382 388 150 email: ContactUs@ dundee.ac.uk www.dundee.ac.uk /admissions /undergraduate	MDSc Prosthodontics MRes Oral Cancer MSc Oral Biology MFOdont Forensic Odontology MRes Cancer Biology MDPH Dental Public Health Research degrees (PhD/MSc): Dental Public Health/Health Services Oral Cancer Clinical Trials Craniofacial Anomalies
Edinburgh Edinburgh Postgraduate Dental Institute University of Edinburgh Lauriston Building Lauriston Place Edinburgh EH3 9HA	Tel: 0131 536 4970 www.dentistry.ed.ac.uk	MSc/Diploma/Certificate Primary Dental Care
Glasgow The University of Glasgow The Fraser Building Hillhead Street Glasgow G12 8QF	Tel: 0141 330 6062 Fax: 0141 330 2961 email: student.recruitment@ glasgow.ac.uk www.glasgow.ac.uk	MSc (Dent. Sci): Fixed & Removable Prosthodontics Oral & Maxillofacial Surgery Endodontics DClin Orthodontics Research degrees available
Lancashire School of Medicine and Dentistry University of Central Lancashire Allen Building Preston PR1 2HE	Tel: 01772 892 400 www.uclan.ac.uk	MSc/PgDip: Oral Surgery Non Surgical Facial Aesthetics for registered healthcare professionals Dental Implantology MSc/PgDip/PgCert: Endodontolgy Periodontology Clinical Restorative Cosmetic Dentistry PgCert: Clinical Dental Technology Studies Commissioning & Dental Advising MSc Prosthodontics

Table 7.1 (*continued*)

Dental school	Contact details	Examples of courses
		BSc (Hons) Dental Studies (Dental Care Professionals) DipOrthTher(RCSE) Dip Orthodontic Therapy Cert. Oral health application of fluoride varnish AdvCert Mentoring in Dental Practice Cert Level 7 Facilitating learning in health care practice
Leeds The University of Leeds Woodhouse Lane Leeds LS2 9JT	Tel: 0113 343 3999 email: admissions@leeds.ac.uk www.leeds.ac.uk	MSc Dental Public Health, 1 year full time MSc Paediatric Dentistry, 2 years full time or 3 years part time Distance learning courses: MSc Restorative Dentistry MSc Implant Dentistry Research degrees: Biomaterials Biomineralisation Craniofacial Biology Dental Public Health Oral and Maxillofacial Surgery Oral Microbiology Orthodontics Paediatric Dentistry Restorative Dentistry Tissue Engineering PhD/Professional Doctorate: Paediatric Dentistry MPhil MDS
Liverpool The University of Liverpool The Foundation Building Brownlow Hill Liverpool L69 7ZX	Tel: 0151 794 2000 Fax: 0151 708 6502 email: ugrecruitment@liv.ac.uk www.liv.ac.uk	Doctorate in Dental Science Orthodontics Endodontics

(*continued overleaf*)

Table 7.1 (*continued*)

Dental school	Contact details	Examples of courses
London Barts and the London School of Medicine and Dentistry Garrod Building Turner Street Whitechapel London E1 2AD	Tel: 020 7882 2240 www.dentistry.qmul.ac.uk	MClinDent: Prosthodontics Oral Medicine MSc Endodontic Practice: Dental Materials Dental Technology Experimental Oral Pathology Dental Science for Clinical Practice PGDip Dental Technology Dental Clinical Sciences Foundation Cert in OHE Research PhD
London King's College London University of London Strand London WC2R 2LS	Tel: 020 7848 5454 Fax: 020 7848 7171 email: prospective@kcl.ac.uk www.kcl.ac.uk	MSc Dental Public Health MSc Paediatric Dentistry
London Eastman Dental Hospital Gray's Inn Road London WC1X 8LD	Tel: 020 3456 1038 www.eastman.ucl.ac.uk	PhD Studentships MSc Restorative Dental Practice MSc Oral Medicine PgCert Dental Sedation and Pain Management PgCert Paediatric Dentistry
London Queen Mary University of London Mile End Road London E1 4NS	Tel: 020 7882 5555 Fax: 020 7882 5500 email: admissions@qmul.ac.uk www.qmul.ac.uk	MClinDent (oral surgery) (periodontology) MSc Implant Dentistry
Manchester The University of Manchester Oxford Road Manchester M13 9PL	Tel: 0161 275 2077 Fax: 0161 275 2106 email: admis- sions@manchester.ac.uk www.manchester.ac.uk	PgDip Control of Pain and Anxiety MSc Prosthodontics MPhil/PhD: Basic Dental Science Cancer Studies Molecular Genetics Stem Cell Biology Biomaterials Science and Dental Technology Dental Public Health/ Community Dentistry PhD (Clin) Dental Science Clinical

Table 7.1 (*continued*)

Dental school	Contact details	Examples of courses
Newcastle Newcastle University King's Gate Newcastle upon Tyne NE1 7RU	Tel: 0191 208 3333 Fax: 0191 222 6143 www.ncl.ac.uk	PGCert Clinical Implant Dentistry PGDip Conscious Sedation MSc Orthodontics MClinDent Restorative Dentistry
Plymouth Peninsula College of Medicine & Dentistry The John Bull Building Tamar Science Park Research Way Plymouth PL6 8BU	Tel: 01752 437 333 Fax: 01752 517 842 email: pcmd-admissions@pcmd.ac.uk www.pcmd.ac.uk	PG Cert, PgDip, Masters: Restorative Dentistry MSc Biomedical Sciences Research Degrees
Sheffield The University of Sheffield Northumberland Road Sheffield S10 2TT	Tel: 0114 222 8030 Fax: 0114 222 8032 www.sheffield.ac.uk	Doctorate in Clinical Dentistry: Endodontics Periodontics Prosthodontics Masters: Dental Materials Science Dental Implantology Dental Public Health Diagnostic Oral Pathology Orthodontics Paediatric Dentistry Social Science and Oral Health Dental Technology

dental school so that you can either contact them directly or view the courses online to decide if they are what you are looking for.

- **Certificate:** Dental Law and Ethics.
- **Cert. Med. Ed.:** Post Compulsory Education.
- **Masters Programmes:** Dental Public Health, Public Health.
- **Doctorate Programmes:** Doctor of Philosophy.
- **DMed Eth:** Medical Ethics.

> **Top Tip:** *Don't argue with a foolish person; you will never win, just walk away*
>
> Shazad Malik

Table 7.2 Royal colleges

College	Contact details	Examples of courses
Royal College of Surgeons of England Faculty of Dental Surgery 35–43 Lincoln's Inn Fields London WC2A 3PE	Tel: 020 7869 6810 Fax: 020 7869 6816 email: fds@rcseng.ac.uk www.rcseng.ac.uk/fds	FDS (Fellow of Dental Surgery) Dip. Primary Care Dip. Special Care Dentistry
Royal College of Surgeons of England Faculty of Dental General Practice (UK) Provides courses and accredits post-registration courses	Tel: 020 7869 6754 www.fgdp.org.uk	Dip. Restorative Dentistry Dip. Membership of the Joint Dental Faculties (MJDF) Cert. Appraisal of Dental Practices Cert. Mentoring in Dentistry Cert. Oral Surgery Cert. Dental Health Services Leadership/ Management
Royal College of Physicians and Surgeons Edinburgh	Tel: 0131 527 1600 www.rcsed.aca.uk	Diploma in Implant Dentistry Dip. Membership in Special Needs Dentistry
Royal College of Surgeons, Ireland 123 St Stephen's Green Dublin	+353 402 2239/2256 facdentistry@rcsi.ie www.rcsi.ie	Fellow of Faculty of Dentistry (FFD)

> *Top Tip:* Keep learning
>
> Derek Richards

Universities

Many of the courses included in Table 7.3 are nonclinical, but they all have relevance to dentistry and dental professional career pathways. They are a very small sample of what is available.

> *Career Highlight:* President of the British Dental Association
>
> Janet Clarke

Other course/programme providers

Please note the list of providers and courses in Table 7.4 is not exhaustive, but merely an example of what is available.

Table 7.3 Universities

University	Contact details	Examples of courses
University of Bedfordshire Department of Clinical Education and Leadership Union Square Luton Bedfordshire LU1 3JU	Tel: 01582 743989 www.beds.ac.uk	PgCert Dental Law and Ethics PgCert Dental Education PgCert Medical Education (Leadership)
University of Kent The Registry Canterbury Kent CT2 7NZ	Tel: 01634 402020 email: admis- sions@midkent.ac.uk www.midkent.ac.uk	Foundation Degree – Advanced Dental Nursing PgCert/PgDip Primary Dental Care Research Skills Clinical Education Leadership and Management Clinical Practice Appraisal
University of Northampton Park Campus Boughton Green Rd Northampton NN2 7AL	Tel: 0800 3582232 www.northampton.ac.uk	Foundation Degree – Dental Nursing
University of Warwick Medical School Coventry CV4 7AL	www.wbs.ac.uk	Cert/Dip/MSc Implant Dentistry MSc Orthodontics MSc Endodontics MSc Restorative & Aesthetic Dentistry
University of Westminster 309 Regent St London W1B 2HW	Tel: 02476 574880 email: d.vogel@westminster .ac.uk www.Westminster.ac .uk/journalism	Medical Journalism BA Honours 1 year
University of Chester Parkgate Rd Chester CH1 4BJ	Tel: 01244 512456 email: postgrad@chester.ac.uk www.chester.ac.uk	PgCert Mastery of Dental Practice Management PgCert/Dip/Msc Cognitive Behavioural Sciences
University of London Kings College London Queen Mary (QMUL) Strand London WC2R 2LS	Tel: 020 7836 5454 www.kcl.ac.uk	LLM (Master of Laws), General, Medical Law PgCert/PgDip/MSc Evidence Based Healthcare
University of Oxford Rewley House 1 Wellington Sq. Oxford OX1 21A	Tel: 01865 286943 email: cpdhealth@conted.ox .ac.uk	MSc Evidence Based Healthcare
Anglia Ruskin University Cambridge and Chelmsford campuses	Tel: 01245 493131 email: pmi@anglia.ac.uk www.anglia.ac.uk/ruskin	PgCert/PgDip/MSc Medical and Healthcare Education

Table 7.4 Other courses/programme providers

Provider	Contact Details	Examples of Courses
National Leadership Academy	Tel: 0113 322 5659 email: leadingcare@leadership academy.nhs.uk www.nationalleadership academy.nhs.uk	NHS Graduate Management Training Scheme Top Leaders programme Edward Jenner Mary Seacole Nye Bevan
Forton Group College Farm Main St Willoughby Warwicshire CV23 8BH	Tel: 0845 0772980 email: info@thefortongroup .com www.thefortongroup .com	Coaching, Leadership, Interview Skills, Mentoring
Jan Laver International Centre for Coaching and Leadership Development Oxford Brookes University Business School Wheatley Campus Oxford OX33 1HX	Tel: 01865 484534 email: jlaver@brookes.ac.uk	Coaching Leadership Development
The Beadle Society of Apothecaries Apothecaries' Hall Black Friars Lane London EC4V 6EJ	Tel: 020 7236 1189 Fax: 020 7329 3177 email: beadle@ apothecaries.org	Diploma in History of Medicine Diploma in Philosophy of Medicine Diploma in Forensic Medical Sciences Diploma in Medical Jurisprudence

> *Career Highlight: Sri Lanka Team Administrator/ Organiser*
> Emma Worrell

Financial investment

Costs vary with the level of the qualification, the length of training and the format of delivery, but the investment is a substantial one in most cases. You should expect to pay over £20 000 for a distance-learning masters programme, for example, generally spread over 3 years.

Other sources of information about courses

- **Dental Schools Council:** www.dentalschoolscouncil.ac.uk.
- **Northern Ireland Medical and Dental Training Agency:** www.nimdta .gov.uk.
- **Royal College of Surgeons (England):** https://www.rcseng.ac.uk/fds /careers-in-dentistry, https://www.rcseng.ac.uk/fds/jcptd/higher-specialist -training/higher-specialist-training (information on higher specialist training documents and the curriculum for each specialty).
- **Faculty of General Dental Practice (UK):** FGDP Career Pathway, http: //www.fgdp.org.uk/_assets/career%20pathway%20step%20by%20step% 20info.pdf.

Useful organisations and networks

- **Committee of Postgraduate Dental Deans and Directors (COPDEND):** www.copdend.org. The Web site gives contact details for all dental deaneries in the United Kingdom. A number of postgraduate deaneries have well established mentoring training programmes and leadership programmes. Some also offer coaching training.
- **Universities and Colleges Admissions Service (UCAS):** www.ucas.com.
- **Coaching and Mentoring Network:** www.coachingnetwork.org.uk.
- **Chartered Institute of Personnel and Development:** www.cipd.co.uk.
- **European Mentoring and Coaching Council:** www.emccouncil.org.
- **Employment National Training Organisation:** www.ento.co.uk.
- **International Coach Federation:** email icfheadquarters@coachfederation .org.

Case studies

It is important to consider the qualifications and training you will need as you progress through your career. However, I think it is also important to hear from people who are actually doing the job you are interested in. In this section I include descriptions from dental professionals of a selection of qualification and training paths they have completed. The individuals have kindly written about their own experiences in gaining specific qualifications. Please be aware that often a range of routes are possible; you might not wish to follow the route described but still want to reach the same destination.

> **Top Tip:** *Beg for forgiveness rather than ask permission*
> Janet Clarke

Certificate in Oral Health Education: Mrs Geraldine Birks

Entry requirements None apart from being a registered dental nurse.

Course content Oral health and anatomy.

Teaching, lesson planning and delivery of oral health education to patients.

Communication, equality and diversity.

Time commitment Part-time course. I commission this post-qualification for Health Education England, Yorkshire & the Humber. Our course runs for one full day per month for 6 months at a hotel venue. Considerable home study is required to meet the learning outcomes necessary for successful completion.

Cost of the course Health Education England, Yorkshire & The Humber supports the dental nurse workforce by heavily subsidising the course (the cost was £150 in 2014). Elsewhere, the cost is usually around £800.

Format Tutored sessions with home study. e-learning options also available.

Top tips A really enjoyable qualification to undertake. Relevant to your work as a dental nurse and easily implemented into practice. It will enhance your CV and give you the opportunity to raise the oral health status of your patients. You will be able to do some real good and enjoy the added responsibility.

I would really recommend dental nurses undertake this qualification as part of their professional development and become extended-duty dental nurses.

Orthodontic therapist: Mrs Sophie Noske

Entry requirements Certificate in dental nursing. It would be helpful if you had a post-registration qualification in orthodontic nursing, but this is not essential.

Course content Principles of orthodontic therapy.

Removable orthodontic appliances.

Fixed orthodontic appliances.

Biomedical sciences, oral biology.

Interdisciplinary working.

Time commitment 1 year full time or 18 months part time. Initial 4-week block + eight study days + workplace training.

Cost of the course £12 500 (2014).

Format Blended seminars, lectures, problem-based learning and projects. In addition, clinical training. Workplace clinical mentor/trainer in an approved orthodontic practice or department with a specialist or consultant orthodontist.

Top tips Go for it – it will change your life.

Make sure you have a supportive trainer who respects your limitations.

Career Highlight: Setting up the National Council of Caldicott Guardians
Janine Brooks

Examiner MJDF: Mr Peter Thornley

Entry requirements A postgraduate qualification. Mentoring experience/ qualification may help. Experience helping with a study group. Equality and diversity training etc.

Course content Usually training is provided by the institution for their examiners. However, a postgraduate certificate of education or similar would help your career progression.

Time commitment Usually two diets per year of 2 days per diet. Time for examiner training: another day or so. Time at home background reading and writing questions.

Cost of the course No cost, but most examiners are voluntary so GDPs lose time in the practice.

Format Training sessions by exam board involve various formats, lectures, role play etc. Small groups for question setting can work well.

Top tips Get involved with a local examination study group first.

Get stuck in – write questions etc. Not many people take an active role, and if you do, you will progress to more senior roles within the faculty.

Honorary Research Fellow: Mr Peter Thornley

Entry requirements A postgraduate dental qualification can help get you started and help you begin to build a network. The Fellowship in General Dental Practice of the FGDP(UK) has a research domain.

Course content Critical appraisal and literature searching skills are very useful, as is some experience writing up research – most MSc courses would include this kind of material.

Time commitment Meetings maybe once every six weeks, time collecting data in the practice, and if you are a co-author can get quite intensive writing up the research.

Cost of the course If you are lucky, you might win a research grant that helps with your project. MSC courses usually cost about £800 per trimester.

Format Lots of different formats. Face to face, distance learning, e-learning.

Top tips Build a network – make contact with interested colleagues in dental schools. Sometimes doing a part-time teaching job at a dental school can help build a network.

Top Tip: Network (everywhere, all the time)
Janine Brooks

Certificate in Dental Radiology: Miss Jackie Arnold

Entry requirements To be working in a dental practice and have access to radiography facilities and patients to be able to complete the practical part of the qualification.

Course content (only a taster of the content is given) Radiation physics. Electromagnetic spectrum.

Background radiation – natural and artificial.

Radiation protection.

Patient identification and consent.

Regulations.

Routine inspection and testing of equipment.

Digital imaging.

Time commitment Part-time attending college 1 day a week and then completing the practical assessment in the dental practice.

Cost of the course £900 (2014).

Format Face to face.

Top tips If you want to improve your job then increase your knowledge.

Tutor: Miss Bal Chana

Entry requirements *Either* Five GCSEs or O-level passes at grade A – C. These must include English language and a biology-based subject (e.g. human biology, dual science). Plus a nationally recognized dental nursing certificate.

Or Five GCSEs or O-level passes at grade A – C. These must include English language and a biology-based subject (e.g. human biology, dual science) Plus any two A-level subjects with grades or predicted grades at A – E.

NVQ Level 3 or equivalent qualifications are accepted as two A-level equivalents; however, these must be in a relevant scientific subject, in addition to the minimum requirement of AS-level in biology or human biology at grade C.

Applicants with equivalent qualifications will be considered (e.g. GNVQ, BTEC, access course), but they must have these in a relevant scientific subject, gained to an appropriate standard.

Degree qualifications are accepted if the applicant has a minimum of an AS-level in biology or human biology at grade C.

Additional nursing qualifications, such as dental radiography or the certificate in oral health education, may also help with your application.

Course content The course is very intense and requires 100% commitment throughout the training. Students will undergo regular formative and summative assessments to progress.

Time commitment All courses are full time.

27-month diploma course: Diploma in dental therapy or diploma in dental hygiene.

3-year BSc course: degree in oral health science or degree in dental therapy and dental hygiene.

Cost of the course Diploma courses are NHS-funded.

Students are required to pay student fees for BSc courses.

Format Face-to-face teaching.

Top tips Core qualities of good communication and listening skills; ability to work in a team; respect for colleagues; integrity; ability to recognise your limitations, as well as those of others. Evidence of manual dexterity is desirable.

> *Top Tip: Do what you do, well*
>
> Bal Chana

Orthodontic Hospital Practitioner: Mr Peter Thornley

Entry requirements There are some training courses around for GDPs with an interest in orthodontics. Some of the orthodontic supply companies put them on and some private providers run good hands-on courses.

Course content Weekends to practice bonding up on typodonts and so on, but you really need a training post where you can practice your new skills in a safe environment.

Time commitment Part time, one session per week for the clinical assistant post.

Cost of the course Weekend courses usually in the region of £350 per day.

Format Lectures and hands on.

Top tips Find a place first where you can get some supervised experience – this is the difficult part. Might be some high street orthodontists who would consider mentoring you.

> *Career Highlight: Therapist of the Year 2006*
>
> Bal Chana

> *The best way to predict your future is to create it*
>
> Peter F. Drucker

How to develop experience

So far, I have covered training and qualifications that you might want to consider as you build your career portfolio. These are important, but there is another dimension to building your portfolio, and that is experience. I would like to complete this chapter with some ideas for how you can develop experience.

Experience comes from doing; that is rather obvious, but we can all do lots of things that help build experience in the areas where we need it. Developing clinical experience is straightforward and familiar to dental professionals. Once you have learnt a new clinical skill, such as implant placement, you need to practice, practice, practice. Working with a more experienced colleague or mentor can help considerably. It helps if they are at the same site as you, so that you can meet up easily and discuss cases. However, with modern technology,

Table 7.5 How to develop nonclinical experience

Skill	How to develop
Leadership	Arrange meetings, take forward a practice policy, prepare for a CQC visit
	Become a local councillor
	Introduce a new system into the practice, such as an electronic record system
	Develop a case discussion group with colleagues
	Shadow a colleague
	Volunteer
Negotiation	Become a member of a committee: BDA, LDC, resident or village hall
	Become a local councillor
	Become part of the Local Dental Professional Group
Quality assurance	Become the practice audit lead or an appraiser
Organisation	Volunteer (dental or non-dental)
	Arrange a study group
	Become treasurer or secretary of a group, dental or non-dental
	Be the organiser of the staff meetings at work
Project management	Volunteer (dental or non-dental)
Presentation skills	Lecture
	Present a case at your staff meeting
	Write an opinion piece for a dental journal or publication
	Support the local provider of dental nurse training and tutor a lecture
Political skills	BDA committee, LDC committee
	Take part in the dental committee at dental school (if you are still a student)
	Become a local councillor
Strategic thinking	Become a magistrate
	Serve on a committee
	Become a school or college governor
Management	Introduce a new procedure into the practice
Listening skills	Become a committee member
	Implement a new policy or procedure
	Arrange a study group
	Mentor someone

this is not essential, and you can successfully work with a more experienced colleague who lives and works at a distance from you.

Developing nonclinical experience can be more of a challenge. I give a few ideas and suggestions in Table 7.5.

> **Top Tip:** *Smiling takes less energy than frowning*
>
> Sophie Noske

Professional associations and other useful addresses

British Association of Dental Nurses. PO Box 4, Room 200 Hillhouse International Business Centre, Thornton-Cleveleys, FY5 4QD. Tel: 01253 338 360. email: admin@badn.org.uk. www.badn.org.uk.

British Dental Association. 64 Wimpole Street, London, W1G 8YS. Tel: 020 7935 0875. www.bda.org.

The British Dental Practice Managers Association. 3 Kestrel Court, Waterwells Business Park, Waterwells Drive, Quedgley, Gloucester, GL2 2AT. Tel: 01452 886 364. www.bdpma.org.uk.

The British Dental Trade Association. Mineral Lane, Chesham, Bucks, HP5 1NL. Tel: 01494 782 873. www.bdta.org.uk.

British Society of Dental Hygiene and Therapy. 3 Kestrel Court, Waterwells Business Park, Waterwells Drive, Quedgley, Gloucester, GL2 2AT. Tel: 01452 886 365. email: enquiries@bsdht.org.uk. www.bsdht.org.uk.

City & Guilds Care, Health and Community. 1 Giltspur Street, London, EC1A 9DD Tel: 020 7294 2800. www.city-and-guilds.co.uk.

Dental Laboratories Association. 44–88 Wollaton Road, Beeston, Nottingham NG9 2NR. Tel: 0115 9254 888. Fax: 0115 9254 800. email: info@dla.org.uk. www.dla.org.uk.

General Dental Council. 37 Wimpole Street, London, W1G 8DQ. Tel: 020 7887 3800. www.gdc-uk.org.

The Dental Technologists Association. 3 Kestrel Court, Waterwells Business Park, Waterwells Drive, Gloucester, GL2 2AT. Tel: 0870 243 0753. www.dta-uk.org.

LearnDirect. PO Box 900, Manchester, M60 3LE. Tel: 0800 100 900. www.learndirect.co.uk.

National Examining Board for Dental Nurses. 110 London Street, Fleetwood, Lancashire, FY7 6EU. Tel: 01253 778 417. email: info@nebdn.org. www.nebdn.org.

Bibliography

Anon. (2014). Dental Business Trends 2013. In: The state of UK Dentistry. *British Dental Journal*, **216**, 51.

Dewey, J. (1916). *Democracy and Education: An Introduction to the Philosophy of Education*. Macmillian: London.

Index

How to Develop Your Career in Dentistry, First Edition. Janine Brooks.
© 2015 John Wiley & Sons, Ltd. Published 2015 by John Wiley & Sons, Ltd.